WEIGHT-LOSS HYPNOSIS

WHAT TO DO WHEN COUNTING CALORIES AND CARBS ISN'T CUTTING IT

PAMELA J. LENO

Difference Press

Washington, DC, USA

Published 2021

DISCLAIMER

Neither the author nor the publisher assumes any responsibility for errors, omissions, or contrary interpretations of the subject matter herein. Any perceived slight of any individual or organization is purely unintentional.

Cover design: Jennifer Stimson

Editing: Natasa Smirnov

Author's photo courtesy of: KMW Photography Olympia WA

ADVANCE PRAISE

"In this book, Pam gives you the tools to change your way of thinking and overcome challenges with your weight along with other things. As you read the book, it will guide you into making positive choices and equip you with tools to help create a mindset to make these changes possible and permanent. Taking the time to read Pam's book has been life-changing. Not only have I shed pounds, but I have learned boundaries and positive ways to cope with any situation. Thank you, Pam, for giving me the tools to create a healthy life. I finally have hope and happiness."

— GINA K

"In *Weight-Loss Hypnosis* Pam uses her own personal life and massive amounts of research and practical use. Pam will guide you on your journey to a happier, healthier lifestyle.

The analogies and stories of "real" people are examples of how to find balance to live life from the inside out. Knowledge is power. Obtaining the knowledge to make life-changing choices is a defining goal of this book, and Pam offers tried and true ways to nurture you toward that goal. You are given encouragement and tools to dig deep into your heart to find your personal answer. Although this book is geared toward weight loss, the information and techniques can help any area of life you wish to improve."

— M. RAY

"Pam's words inspire readers for more as she will reach many who have failed over and over on their dieting roller coaster. Techniques, tips, common sense, and facts are rolled into a simple short, condensed guide, easy to follow and understand. She has given all of us the tools for reference in her new book *Weight-Loss Hypnosis, What to Do When Counting Calories and Carbs Isn't Cutting It.*"

— REBECCA C

"I thoroughly enjoyed reading Pam's book, *Weight-Loss Hypnosis*. It is very applicable to the increasing complex stressors that are happening today. She has taken complicated scientific information and simplified it for our own common use. I personally found it helpful to put her main self-help techniques on a four-by-six card to remind me to use them, thus improving my mental and physical wellbeing. I have plenty of patients that have and will benefit from the knowledge and techniques presented in this book."

— ROBERT N

"For anyone contemplating weight-loss surgery I would read this book and use the tools. Hypnotherapy is life-changing. This works! I have done every diet including bypass and Pam's book has taught me how food affects me and how to resolve issues that were causing me to overeat. I am on the road to recovery, and this is how you can resolve your past issues of self-medicating with food."

— DEBBIE A

CONTENTS

To Bob Nooney, my rib.

You believed in me and stood beside me through the many ideas, actions, and thoughts that brought me to writing this book. Thank you.

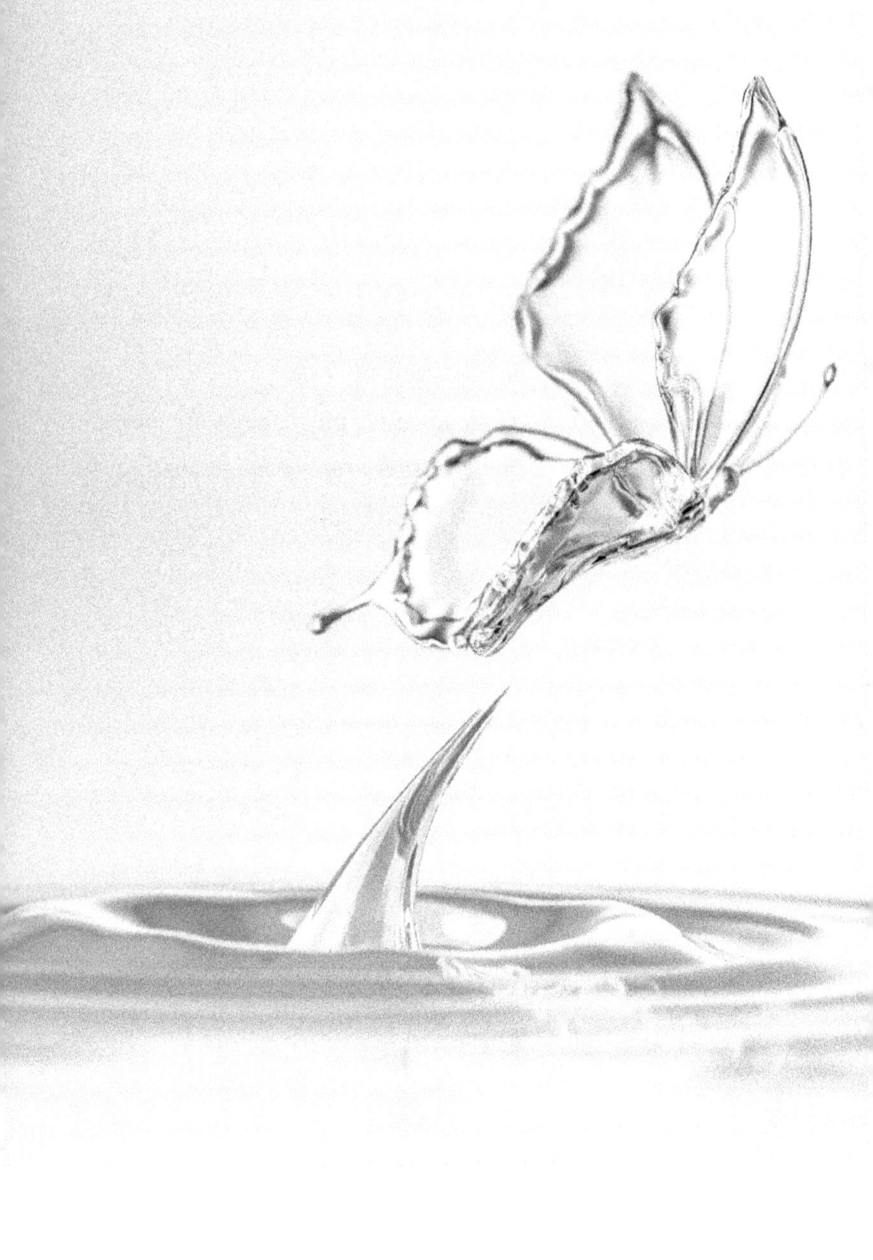

1

IT IS NEVER ABOUT THE DIET

Gina was so looking forward to Thanksgiving. Her two older kids were flying in and the whole family was going to sit down for a nice meal. The very idea of sharing a meal with her two adult kids, her moody teen, and her husband warmed her heart. If she could make all their favorite dishes just right, if she could fill their bellies with pure, unadulterated enjoyment, maybe she could fill their hearts with it, too?

Gina was having a hard time in her second marriage. Her husband was often disrespectful and demeaning to her. She was wondering if she should even stay in the marriage. Her grown-up kids were off leading their own lives and that wasn't helping her feel fulfilled either. So, she fell into her usual holiday frenzy thinking one feast can make it all better.

A feast. That's when the guilt started to kick in: "Yeah, Gina, plan to stuff yourself as usual. No wonder you can't lose the extra seventy-five pounds. Calorie counting did not work. Carb counting did not work. Grinding yourself into a puddle of sweat at the gym did not work. Atkins, keto, vegan – nothing ever works because you are just a fatty who loves to eat. You are out of control. What is wrong with you? "

Gina shared her spiraling with a coworker who recommended she come and see me. And luckily she did. Our first conversation was inundated with feelings of hopelessness and overall misery. Gina's summary of her problem went something like this: "What's the point? Sooner or later, I'm going to fail. I always have. Sometimes it happens after a month, sometimes after a year, but the pounds always come back and usually with a vengeance. Lately, they don't even fall off for a little while." Gina felt defeated. Sounds familiar, right?

It is not your fault that you are overweight and keep wanting to soothe yourself by putting something in your mouth. We are taught this as soon as we leave the womb. When we have a wet diaper, are hungry, or express any kind of discontent, we have something shoved into our mouths – a nipple, a pacifier, a bottle. And then, as we mature a bit, we associate food with relief when we feel bad.

It goes like this: "Oh, Gina it's okay that you lost the soccer game. Let's go get some ice cream. That will make you feel better." Sound familiar? Or then there is the celebration part: "Wow, you did such a great job on that test! Let's go get pizza and celebrate." You can see how this creates a recipe for weight gain. You associate food with feeling better because that is what has been planted in your subconscious mind from the time you drew your first breath.

Then there are the holidays. "Let's all get together and eat until we can't move." Who hasn't experienced the famous Thanksgiving hangover? This, too, is associated with feeling better because everyone else is doing it. You share the groans of disbelief over how tight your pants feel all of the sudden. You belong.

However, if you think about it for a second, these warm and fuzzy feelings don't come from food at all. It's about companionship, caring, family, *love*. These are the real soothers. What really comforted you was the fact that someone cared. Someone wanted to take you for ice cream; someone wanted to celebrate with pizza and that was really the comfort for you. At Thanksgiving or other holidays, you are surrounded by people who care about you (hopefully). So yes, take a minute to process this and accept that this is not your fault. You were (are) seeking comfort and love. You will see later how common this is and learn how to understand what your emotions are trying to tell you and how *not* to feed them but actually understand them. Feeling emotions is nature's way of experiencing life. Think what life would be like if we didn't have love, happiness, enthusiasm, hope.

All emotions are good. Both pleasant and unpleasant. I am sure you understand what pleasant emotions are – happiness, hope, joy, love. But what about the unpleasant ones? Things like anger, boredom, sadness, loneliness, fear, stress, guilt, unworthiness? They too have a message for you. All these "yucky" feelings are trying to tell you there is a need, want, or desire that is not being met. Anger is trying to tell you that something is unfair either to you or someone you care about. Boredom is telling you there is a lack of something interesting or it is covering for some other emotion you do not want to feel, like loneliness. Fear is often the root of all other negative emotions. It is a call to action. However, we often freeze instead. Guilt simply is indicating an action that was taken that was unfair to others. All of these emotions are needing something changed to feel better. However, putting something in your mouth will not remove the emotion or change the unmet need, want, or desire. In fact, feeding your emotions will actually make you feel worse. It might give you a moment's pleasure, but then the guilt, self-hatred, or regret flow in, and you've now doubled the discomfort you were seeking relief from. There will be valuable tools for you to use instead of eating your emotions following soon. Yes, something that will actually work.

HOW COULD THIS BE ANY DIFFERENT THAN ALL THE THINGS I HAVE TRIED BEFORE?

Gina began hypnotherapy and applying the education I gave her on what she was eating and how it was actually affecting her body. She practiced the tools I taught her regularly. Today she has reached her weight loss goal. She has begun a new career that she loves, and practices self-hypnosis daily. She has set boundaries with her husband, and he is now respectful and genuinely kind. Gina is happier than she has been in her life! Her family and friends all want to know what she is doing. I am here to tell you: you, too, can do this!

I am sure you are wondering how this will be any different than what you have tried before. I understand. Most of my clients come to me with the same query on their minds. This is a new and completely different process that involves science, spirituality, and self-hypnosis. That is new. We will look into the science of the body, the connection with your own personal spirituality, and the technique of self-hypnosis. – the three pillars of success of my hundreds of clients.

Regular diets do not work because they have you completely focused on food at all times. Plus, there is usually a beginning and an end. But what do you do after that? They will work temporarily but you are working completely with just your brain and willpower, and I think you will agree – it is exhausting! Your willpower will let you down, then you feel bad. This is the eat-feel bad-eat cycle that is sabotaging your success. Education on how food affects your hormones, how sugar is addictive, and why exercise is not an effective way to lose weight will begin to make so much sense!

WHY EXERCISE ALONE DOESN'T WORK

To burn just one pound of fat you must run twenty-six miles. A pound of fat is around 3,500 calories. Yep, you would have to run twenty-six miles to expend that many calories through exercise. So, it is very difficult to exercise and lose weight. Especially if you do not change what you are putting in your mouth. Exercise is important for overall health, and I highly recommend it. However, it will discourage you if that is how you try to burn fat. Especially if you are obese or morbidly obese with a BMI of more than thirty due to the stress movement creates on your joints. Did you know that when you walk and/or run, the pressure on your feet is four to six times your body weight? Let's break that down. You weigh 200 pounds. Multiply by six and that is 1,200 pounds of pressure on your feet, ankles, knees. No wonder your feet hurt at the end of the day. Over time, the joints will wear down and that is when chronic pain creeps in. One of the comments I've heard over and over is, "Since I lost thirty pounds, my knees don't hurt anymore." One of my clients avoided knee surgery simply by reducing his body weight.

Now you know how far you must run to burn

one pound of body fat. My clients who use energy-expenditure devices, like Fitbit or Apple Watch, are amazed by how few calories are expended with an hour of movement. I hear often, "Man I rode my bike for an hour and only used 150 calories!" Yep. So, you see, it is very difficult to exercise to lose weight.

Now, consider one cup of ice cream – just plain vanilla. That's 274 calories. Remember that hour on the bike? That's only 150 calories spent. So, are you willing to ride a bike for two hours for that one cup of ice cream? When you look at it from this perspective, it really begins to make sense that what you are putting in your mouth has more weight. (Pun intended!) As you continue to read this book it will become even clearer to you how the changes you make really do count.

My dream for you is that for the first time in your life you will have the ability to truly be successful – not only in losing weight, but in reconnecting with your inner light and turning it back on. You will feel lighter physically, mentally, and spiritually. This is a wonderful way to live. I can help you get there.

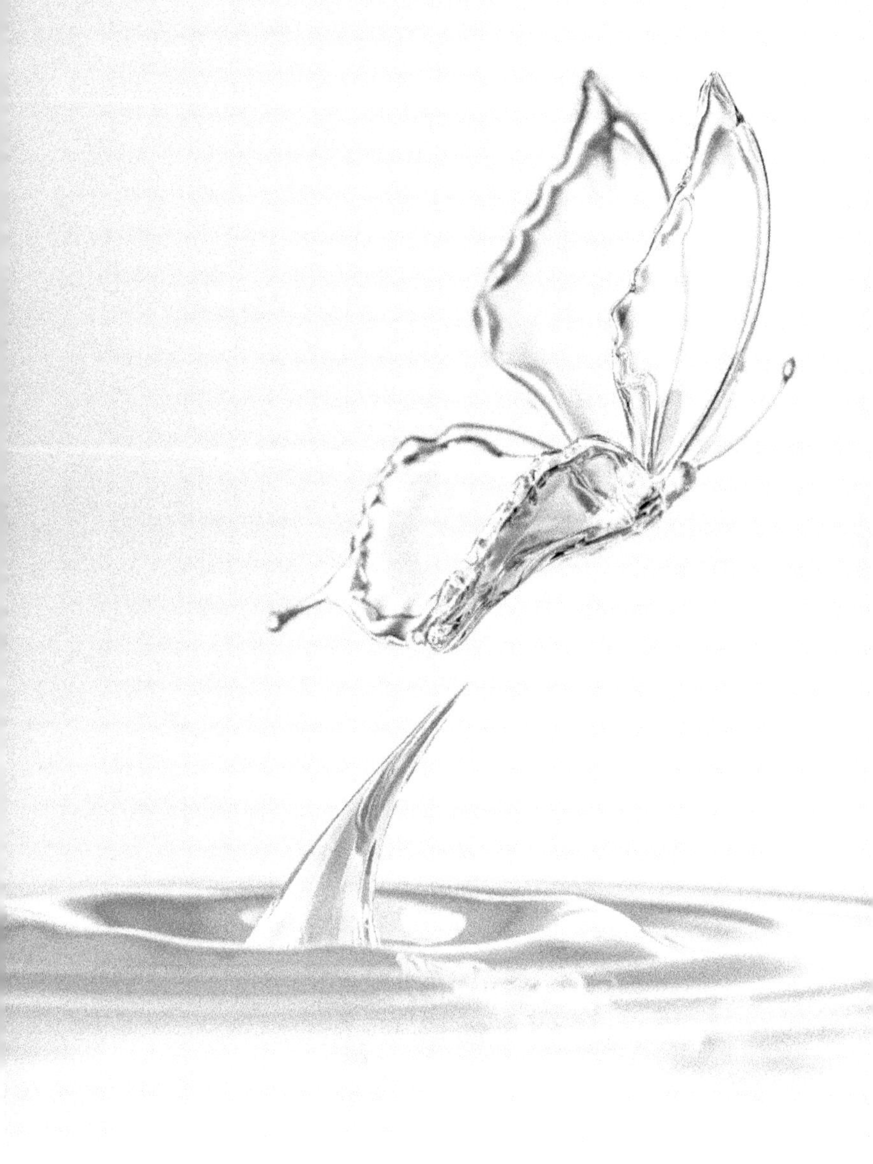

2

WHO AM I AND WHY SHOULD YOU TRUST ME?

My career in wellness began a long time ago. I worked in the fitness industry for thirty years as an aerobics instructor. Yes, Jane Fonda was my mentor – leg warmers and all! When I began there were no certifications or training. We just danced and jumped around. After a few years, the American Council on Exercise (ACE) actually created a curriculum and test for instructors to help educate and prevent injury. I passed and continued forward instructing at little fitness clubs around the area I lived in Oregon at the time. Later I married and had two children. After divorce number one, I moved to western Washington, near Seattle. I found the Washington Athletic Club in downtown Seattle and began instructing there. Eventually I directed the complete group fitness program and developed and implemented many new and creative classes. We introduced yoga, Pilates, and group cycling, which at that time were not prevalent in the fitness industry. At one point I overcame my fear of water by teaching myself to swim and participated in a triathlon and became a triathlon coach. Interestingly enough, I would beat people up in my classes expecting them to lose weight. It didn't work as I am sure you already know. After 18 years at the WAC and divorce number two, I left the fitness industry.

After years of being a drill sergeant and expecting people to lose weight by pushing them harder and harder in boot camp class, I turned to education and supplemented diets. Since I was no longer working out three to four hours a day or teaching classes in the fitness arena, I also gained a bunch of weight because then I was sitting at a desk for hours. It was time for me to implement what I had learned on myself!

In 2011, I met Dr. Robert (Bob) Nooney through an online dating app. I lived in Lake Stevens, Washington, and he lived in Olympia, Washington. After some time, it became evident that we wanted to be together. I had more flexibility, so I moved to Olympia, Washington, and changed the direction of my career. I started my wellness clinic in Olympia, Washington – Ideal Wellness NW – and with Bob's help I continued my education on how food actually affects our bodies, our hormones, and disease.

I teamed up with Bob and together we implemented a partial meal replacement that really did help clients and patients lose weight and get off many medications. We also added a registered dietician to our protocol with a whole foods option. These "diets" worked because we also taught a lifestyle change that actually could be followed and after losing weight , our clients maintain the achieved results. The problem with this is that the beliefs, thoughts, and old behaviors seemed to creep back in and many of our "successful" clients were returning a few years later right where they started. What was going on?

I decided that life coaching was the key and became certified in both Law of Attraction (LoA) and high-performance coaching. Both valuable but took a lot of work on behalf of my clients and most did not want to put the effort in that I was asking. Coaching requires self-reflection, goal setting, daily tasks, reading, and courage. Most of my clients just did not have the motivation to really use the tools I was teaching them. One day – and I believe, by divine intervention – hypnotherapy came across my radar. I really don't even remember how, but it was an instant knowing that this was something I wanted to look into. I became certified in LoA hypnotherapy. LoA is working with the concept "what you think about, you create." This type of hypnotherapy resulted in helping my clients feel better and understand what they are thinking and doing is attracting the life they are leading. It was good but not good enough. This technique taught me how to induce hypnosis and did a lot of direct suggestion but felt like there was something missing.

Next, I found Erika Flint at Cascade Hypnosis in Bellingham, Washington, while looking for a noise-cancelling headset. (Divine intervention, ya think!? Amazing the things that come up when you Google!) Erika is an award-winning hypnotist, author, and certified instructor of 5-PATH Hypnosis and 7th Path Self-Hypnosis. These programs were designed by Cal Banyan, MA, board-certified hypnotherapist, certified instructor of hypnotherapy, and supervisor at the Banyan Hypnosis Center for Training and Services. 5-PATH and 7th Path are hypnotherapy process's that build upon each session with outcomes for my clients that I had not seen before as well as teaching me self-hypnosis.

Self-hypnosis has been a life-changer for me. I struggled with decision-making, self-confidence, trust, and faith. I was trying to do everything with willpower and push. Life was not flowing easily. I was tired. Now that I am truly connected and trust my Higher Power, this new way of living has filled my life with peace, confidence, faith, calmness, and joy. I practice self-hypnosis daily and connect with my Higher Power. And the best part is that I learned to teach this method of self-care to my clients and the results are finally all-encompassing and permanent.

Meredith, for example, came to me having failed at another diet. She couldn't seem to get her eating under control and was considering going on medication for depression. Her blood sugar and cholesterol were elevated, and she was on blood pressure medication. Through the education and understanding of how the foods she was eating were affecting her hormones and health, she began to change what she was putting in her mouth. She practiced the self-hypnosis I taught her in earnest and really began to enjoy the time she was giving to herself to heal and regain her health. As a bonus, she underwent some major dental surgery using her self-hypnosis to remain calm and collected during the ten-hour procedure in the dentist chair. (Her dentist is now a client, too!) Today she is healthier by far and is enjoying her life from a place of peace and joy. Her energy and vitality are so much higher. She has lost the weight and is keeping it off with the new healthy lifestyle she adopted.

Since adding hypnosis and self-hypnosis to our clinic menu, we have helped hundreds if not thousands of people lose weight and keep it off successfully, and also improve their lives in numerous other ways as well. However, I realized there are only so many hours in the day and, consequently, only so many people I can work with. And I, once again, wanted to do more. (Do you see a pattern?) So here I am today writing a book to help you, my dear reader, regain your healthy body, mind, and spirit. With the understanding you will receive, and the practices taught in this book, you will regain the love of life and yourself again.

Hope and possibility are yours.

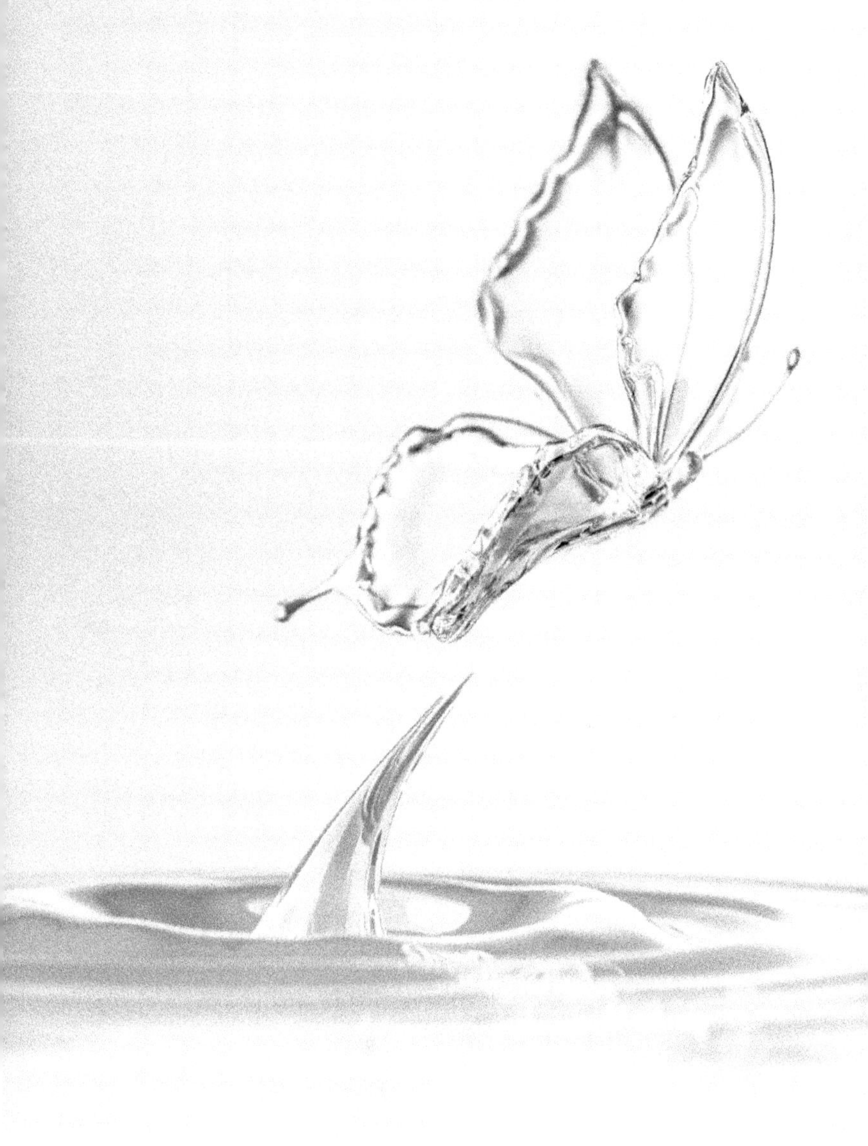

3

READY TO GET CONTROL OF YOUR LIFE?

I recommend that you, first, read this book to the end and then go back and reread the education techniques and practices to apply to your daily life. Please know, as you read this book, many of the ideas shared may not make complete sense until you finish all the chapters. So, I am going to ask you to bear with me and read on.

Here is a summary of what you can expect to walk away with after each chapter.

In Chapter 4, you will understand how certain foods affect your hormones and why that is so important.

In Chapter 5, we will dive into sugar. Well, not literally, but you will learn how the food industry is creating an unspoken epidemic of obesity and related disease – all the things they do *not* want you to know. For example, you'll discover how sugar is hidden in the food you are eating and the addictiveness of sugar. For those of you with the mind of a scientist, references to studies and research that back this information will be included.

In Chapter 6, I will teach you about stress. You will understand the hormones released during stress and their effect on weight gain and loss. You will learn how untreated or uninterrupted stress hormones affect your health – mentally and physically. Stress is the silent killer that is never listed on a death certificate. We will bring together the trifecta of out-of-control eating: obesity, sugar, and stress. Then you will receive your first four mind-blowing techniques to reduce/ eliminate stress and regain inner peace in a matter of minutes – unwind technique, vagus nerve relaxation, the three yawns method, and access to a relaxation recording.

In Chapter 7, you will understand the gut, heart, and brain connection – how they communicate and how you can actually control the coherence between all three for peace and calmness in your life. With practice, you can literally self-soothe without food!

You will walk away with the Heart Breathing™ practice from the HeartMath™ Institute.

In Chapter 8, you will also understand how very important what you are thinking is and how your thoughts actually affect you physically through cellular vibration. You will actually experience just how powerfully your thoughts affect your body's reaction to them. I will also teach you a brain hack called "Toss the Thought" to reframe self-destructive thinking and reignite your internal cellular vibration for health and vitality.

In Chapter 9, I will introduce you to the long-awaited *self-hypnosis*! You will learn what declarations are, what the purpose of the declarations are, and how to use them daily for your success.

Next, in Chapter 10, you will learn a powerful future progression self-hypnosis technique that will allow you to visualize and feel yourself successful, healthy, and vibrant, plus a link to a guided audio only available to people who have read this book!

Chapter 11 is about what to expect and how to measure your success – physically, mentally, and spiritually.

I'd be remiss if I didn't add a cautionary tale or two. In Chapter 12, I will present some common obstacles that will come up for you in this process and how to understand and navigate them.

Finally, before it's time to say goodbye, I will explain how you can advance on this new journey and continue to grow!

No time like the present. Let's get you your life back!

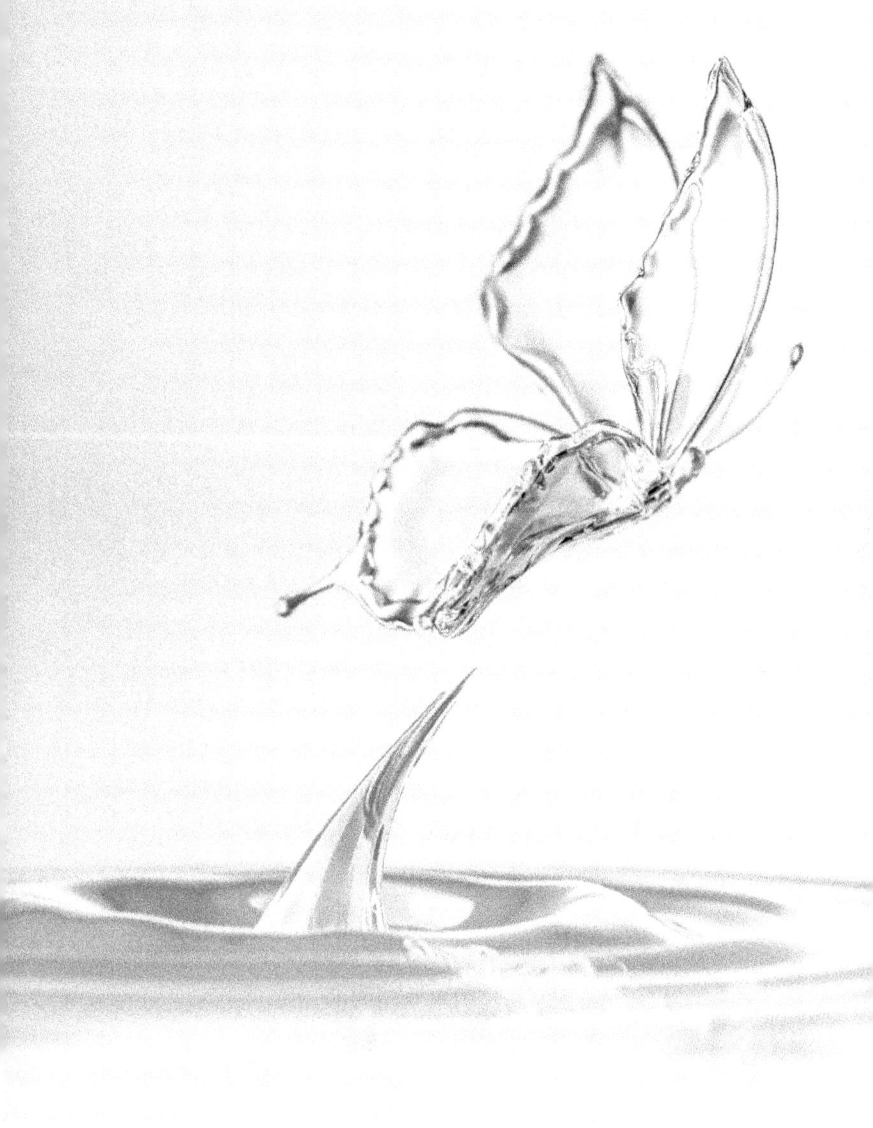

4

FOOD FOR THOUGHT

It is interesting to think about food as fuel for our bodies instead of comfort. Understanding how the food you eat affects your hormones and your health is the gateway to weight loss and better health. All macronutrients (protein, fats, and carbohydrates) affect your hormones when consumed.

Let's consider a common meal choice like a sandwich. A sandwich typically consists of meat, cheese, bread, and a few veggies like lettuce, tomatoes, etcetera.

Meat is protein. Our bodies are made up of mostly protein and water so protein is a very important part of our muscles, skin, and organs. Eating protein provides your body with amino acids which are used to produce specific hormones, like estrogen, insulin, and thyroid hormones (to name a few).

Healthy individuals need at least 0.8 grams of protein per kilogram of body weight per the National Academy of Medicine's (NAM) Dietary Reference Intake. This NAM level is considered to be a *minimum level* for preventing muscle loss. For long-term muscle, metabolic, and overall health, 1 to 1.6 grams of protein per kilogram of body weight is a smarter daily goal to aim for. An easy way to remember this is about half your body weight in grams of protein. For example, a 150-pound woman would need to consume about 70 to 110 grams of protein per day. That's approximately 25 to 35 grams of protein in each meal, if you eat three meals per day. For a woman who's regularly engaging in physical activity, aim for the higher end of this range. Too little protein can result in muscle loss, which cuts strength. Loss of muscle slows metabolism since your muscle is your calorie-burning machine. You may notice weakness, brittle hair and nails, and even hair loss. Lack of protein can even result in loss of bone strength and a weakened immune system. Protein is a vital macronutrient that our bodies need.

Cheese is fat. Fat is essential for all hormone

production. It is important to understand that fat is needed for good brain function, serotonin, and balanced estrogen. Healthy fats include olive oil, avocados, wild-caught fish, coconut oil, etcetera. The dietary reference intake (DRI) for fat in adults is 20 percent to 35 percent of total calories from fat. That is about 44 grams to 77 grams of fat per day if you eat 2,000 calories per day. It is recommended to eat more of some types of fats, like the ones listed above because they provide health benefits. If you eat less than 2,000 calories per day, that amount will need to be adjusted. Healthy fat helps your body absorb vitamins. Healthy fats support cell growth, wound healing plus brain and eye health. Healthy fats help with bowel movements and toxin elimination.

The bottom line when it comes to balanced hormones and fat consumption is to focus on healthy fats and to eliminate damaged fats like vegetable oils, margarine, shortening, and other processed and packaged foods. The body needs fat to function and to make hormones plus keeps your hair shiny, nails strong and skin moisturized. So, don't be afraid to add healthy fats to your diet. With subtle, yet effective changes, your hormones and overall health can greatly benefit, and you may even notice your energy levels, mood, hair, and skin improve, too!

Then, we have veggies. *Yes!* Vegetables are a huge contributor to our hormone balance because the fiber, water, and nutrients help balance our blood sugar, maintain gut harmony, assist in toxin release, and increase antioxidants, all while tasting delicious. When blood sugars are too high from overconsumption of carbohydrates, they can fall sharply and make you feel lightheaded, lethargic, and craving more carbohydrates. If your gut flora or balance is out of wack due to poor eating habits, it cannot create the healthy feelings you desire. That can result in acid reflux and brain fog. Vegetables contain enzymes and fiber which contribute to healthy gut flora. Eating seven to eight servings of an array of raw and cooked vegetables helps to keep us feeling full, increasing our energy levels, and contributing to maintaining a healthy weight and hormonal balance. However, eating too many starchy vegetables – like potatoes, peas, and carrots – can actually contribute to weight gain. It is important to understand the nutrition of the veggies you are eating simply by Googling "nutrition of (whatever vegetable you wish to understand)".

For example, the nutritional panel for a serving of **broccoli** is:

- Calories: 31
- Water: 89 percent
- Protein: 2.5 grams
- Carbs: 6 grams
- Sugar: 1.5 grams
- Fiber: 2.4 grams
- Fat: 0.4 grams

On the other hand, a serving of **potato** is:

- Calories: 168
- Fat: 0 grams
- Protein: 5 grams
- Carbs: 37 grams
- Fiber: 4 grams
- Sodium: 24 milligrams
- Vitamin C: 37 percent of the RDI
- Vitamin B6: 31 percent of the RDI

There is a significant difference in the calories and carbs, as you can see.

But I want to draw your attention to carbohydrates most of all, and how they affect the master hormone – **insulin.** When this hormone is out of balance, it takes a toll on all other hormones.

Let's look at the two slices of bread in your sandwich. Let's say the carbohydrate load in those two slices of plain wheat bread equals 65 grams of carbohydrate. Each 4 grams of carbohydrate equal one teaspoon of sugar, so there are 16.25 teaspoons of sugar in those two pieces of bread. When those grams of carbohydrates enter your bloodstream upon digestion, your pancreas releases the hormone insulin to move that energy from the bloodstream into your muscle so you can use it for movement. There is a factor of fiber, but to keep this as simple as possible and not create a nutrition program, we will look just at the carbs. Now let's say you then have a potato with your dinner. One 3.5-ounce potato has 26 grams of carbohydrate now total for these two meals is 91 grams of carbohydrates or 22.75 teaspoons of sugar. That is too much for most bodies to use on an average day of sitting at your desk. When this occurs continuously over days, months, and years, your body regularly creates too much insulin and your cells become resistant to the hormone. Then your pancreas becomes frantic because the cells are not absorbing the energy and it creates more insulin. Being, also, the fat-storage hormone, insulin must then put that energy somewhere and that is when it lands in your fat cell.

The other issue here is when there is too much insulin in the body, it affects many other hormones. For instance, too much insulin tells the kidneys to retain water and your arterial blood pathways to thicken thus presenting as hypertension or high blood pressure. It tells the ovaries to produce more male hormones and can present as polycystic ovarian syndrome or PCOS. Too much sugar feeds cancer cells. Too much sugar can burn out the pancreas from overwork and lead to diabetes. There is more but I think you get the picture without me laying out the umpteen medical side-effects of too-high carbohydrate intake. Just knowing that insulin is the master hormone and affects the other fifty hormones your body produces is enough to take a look at how you are doing.

At one point in history, we needed that much fuel to work in the fields, to hunt for our food, to travel from mountain to plane, and let's face it, a sandwich is easy, travels well, and meets all the macronutrient needs. Potatoes are easy to grow, store well, and can go a long way in feeding a family. I understand and was raised on a hard-working farm. When you are young you will expend the energy from those types of food easily. Have you ever observed a four-year-old? They run everywhere they go! They never stop! They need that energy to grow and move. As adults, unless you are an athlete, we just don't move that much so that immediate energy from carbohydrates is just not necessary as much as it used to be.

In this chapter, we covered the basics you need to understand and build on. In the next chapter, we will zero in on one particular food and its effects on your body, mind, and emotions. So, as promised in Chapter 3, let's dive into sugar.

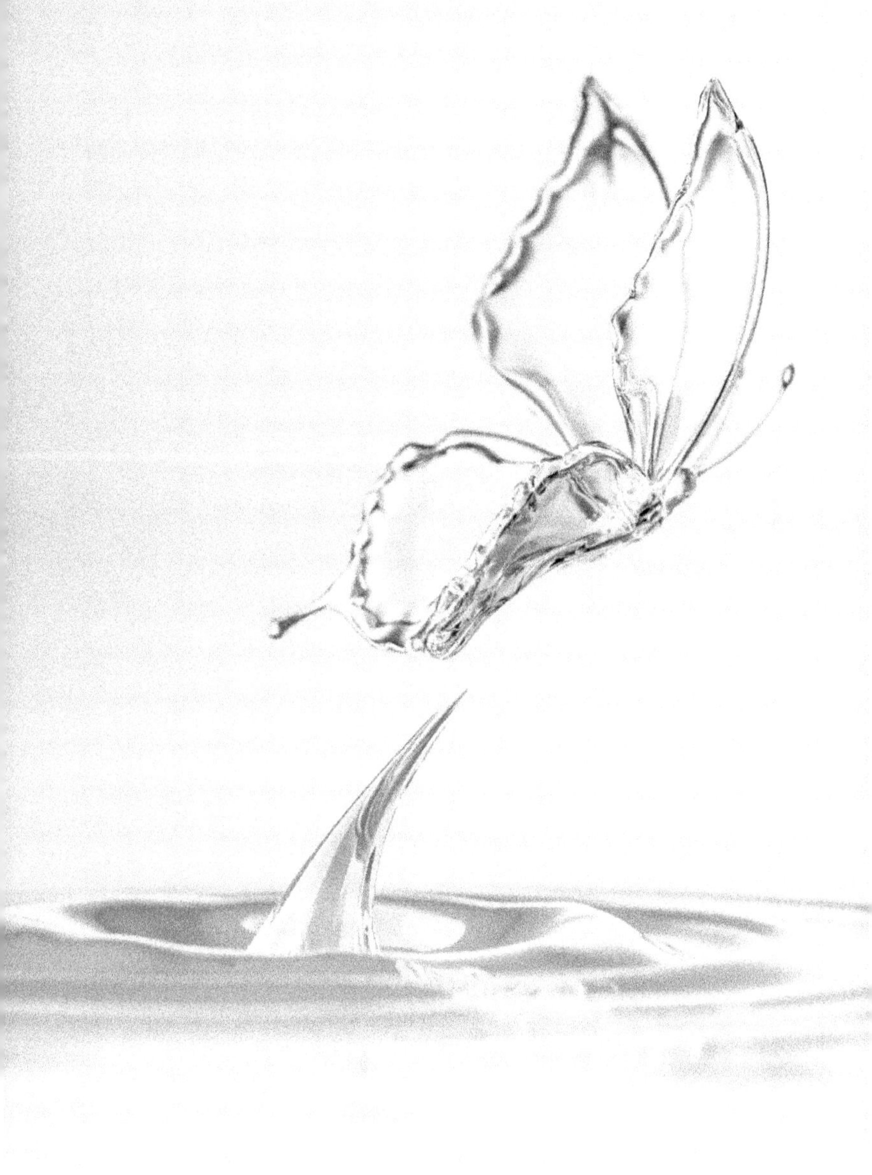

5

SUGAR AND ALL ITS FAVORITE HIDING PLACES

I know you probably know that sugar is not good for you. But do you know why?

According to research, sugar is actually addictive. In an article published in *Scientific American,* Rachel Dvoskin shares, "If the alarming statistics surrounding the so-called obesity epidemic have not convinced you of the dangers of a sugar-packed diet, a new study might have you thinking twice. Rats given a choice between highly sweetened water and intravenous cocaine overwhelmingly favored the sugary tasty beverage. Their preference was just as intense whether the drink was sweetened with saccharin or sugar."

This finding was reported recently by graduate student Magalie Lenoir and her colleagues at the

University of Bordeaux in France. Though researchers are reluctant to generalize, results of several studies confirm that, for some people, sweets could be as pleasurable and addictive as habit-forming drugs. The biggest issue with the modern-day diet is that, unlike in the past, sugar is *everywhere*. We are, therefore, overstimulating our sweet receptors in the brain, which can lead to loss of self-control and an increased risk of addiction. A separate study reported that rats become dependent on sugar and exhibit classic symptoms of withdrawal, both behavioral and neurochemical.

So, how does this relate to you and why is the food industry putting sugar in everything? If you eat foods laced with sugar, chances are you will purchase it again based on the above research. A great marketing idea, wouldn't you agree?

Sugar is added to 80 percent of the food on store shelves. It is a preservative, and the food industry wants the longest shelf-life possible.

Here is an example of something that might surprise you. Take a look at the ingredients of Campbell's vegetable soup:

Beef broth (water, beef stock), carrots, potatoes, tomato paste, peas, pasta (wheat flour, egg white), *sugar*, corn, potato *starch*, green beans, barley, salt, celery, canola or soybean oil, monosodium glutamate, cabbage, dehydrated onions, yeast extract, hydrolyzed protein (soy, corn, wheat), flavor, spices, caramel.

Why do you need sugar in vegetable soup? A healthy option, right? Also, potatoes, carrots, peas, corn, pasta, and barley are all carbohydrates.

Reading labels is an eye-opening experience once you understand what carbohydrate in excess is doing to you and how it is affecting your health and your weight.

Let's take Gina from our first chapter. Some of the items she was eating on a regular basis were oatmeal, toast, rice cakes, sandwiches, potatoes, popcorn, potato chips, and crackers. Over and over, these items eaten in excess created an overweight, depressed, unhappy human.

The other thing the food industry doesn't want you to know is the falsehood of particular scientific research that supposedly linked fat to heart disease, not sugar. Once again, check this out.

The documents in question are five decades old, but the larger issue is of the moment, as Marion Nestle notes in a commentary in an issue of JAMA Internal Medicine.

"Is it really true that food companies deliberately

set out to manipulate research in their favor? Yes, it is, and the practice continues. In 2015, the New York Times obtained emails revealing Coca-Cola's cozy relationships with sponsored researchers who were conducting studies aimed at minimizing the effects of sugary drinks on obesity. Even more recently, the Associated Press obtained emails showing how a candy trade association funded and influenced studies to show that children who eat sweets have healthier body weights than those who do not."

So funding to achieve results on research is quite the fool's way of controlling what we are told, what we believe, and how we operate. Kind of shocking, right?

There is one more very strong point I want to make when it comes to research. There is research that indicates the possibility of high levels of insulin (caused by too much sugar) contribute to cancer-cell growth.

Cancer experts say sugar itself can drive cancer. One such expert is noted cancer researcher Lewis Cantley, PhD, director of the Meyer Cancer Center at Weill Cornell Medicine in New York. Cantley thinks some cancers may start with high levels of insulin, the hormone that controls the amount of sugar in your blood. He says his research shows that "having high levels of insulin is likely to drive cancer. And what drives insulin levels is sugar." Cantley is an American cell biologist and biochemist who has made significant advances to the understanding of cancer metabolism.

Is it all making sense to you now?

NATURAL FOODS AND THE GLYCEMIC INDEX

Having read the previous sections, you might be thinking, "Fine, I'll just steer clear of packaged and processed goods, and I'll be fine, right?" Unfortunately, no! Let's look at "natural" foods and how they can also affect the sugar in your blood stream. You have been taught that fruit is good. After all, the food pyramid suggests two to four servings per day. Let's examine that a bit further. One serving of a banana contains 27 grams of carbohydrates. Using our calculation above you now know that is 6.75 teaspoons of sugar. Then add that to your healthy Raisin Bran and voila – a whopping additional 47 grams of carbohydrates. Ahem, that is 11.75 teaspoons of sugar. Your total sugar intake for just breakfast is then 18.5 teaspoons. Research says you should shoot for 6 teaspoons per day if you're a woman and 9 if you're a man. Yet most people in the U.S. eat about 22 per day. That's 130 pounds of sugar each year. Can you see where this is going? Would you sit down and eat eighteen to twenty teaspoons of sugar? Nope. And this is not even adding the additional carbohydrates throughout the day and the suggested two to four servings. Can you see what is happening? Again, your poor pancreas is working like crazy to get those energy particles out of your bloodstream, yet there is no more room so it must put it into that lovely fat cell that is so ready to accept and store this energy for you for future use. So yes, you can gain weight from fruit. The problem is we continually consume more energy than we are using, and it is just building up, pound by pound. Don't get me wrong, fruit does have its good sides. It is natural, meaning over time, it will rot. That is real food. It has vitamins, minerals, and fibers. Processed foods like potato chips, candy, etcetera, have years of shelf life. Some fruit is absolutely good for you, but can you see why two to four servings a day might be overkill? This prompts me to explain the importance of the glycemic index.

GLYCEMIC INDEX

What is "glycemic index" and how can it help? There are tons of glycemic index charts on the internet. Just Google and you will find one. My goal in this paragraph is to explain what the glycemic index is and how it can help you achieve and maintain weight loss. Here is an explanation of what the glycemic index is used for. Remember that blood glucose equals blood sugar.

According to Wikipedia, "a glycemic index is a number from zero to 100 assigned to a food, with pure glucose (sugar) arbitrarily given the value of 100, which represents the relative rise in the blood glucose level two hours after consuming that food."

For example, watermelon has a glycemic index of seventy-two (remember that pure sugar is 100) whereas asparagus has a glycemic index of fifteen. You can see how that would affect your energy in the blood, the speed of use it would require, and how it would be stored as fat based on what you learned previously. I don't want to overwhelm you here by listing data easily accessible on the internet. However, I think it is a great idea to familiarize and perhaps shock yourself with the glycemic index of the food you're currently eating and how it can be contributing to your weight gain or loss. This knowledge will empower you to make different choices in the future.

Knowledge and awareness are what this chapter is all about. Read the labels. Be mindful of what and how much you're putting in your mouth. It will be shocking at first, perhaps even frustrating. But trust me, it gets easier and stressing about it will not help. I share more on the role of stress in weight gain and how you can stop this from affecting you in the next chapter. So, read on!

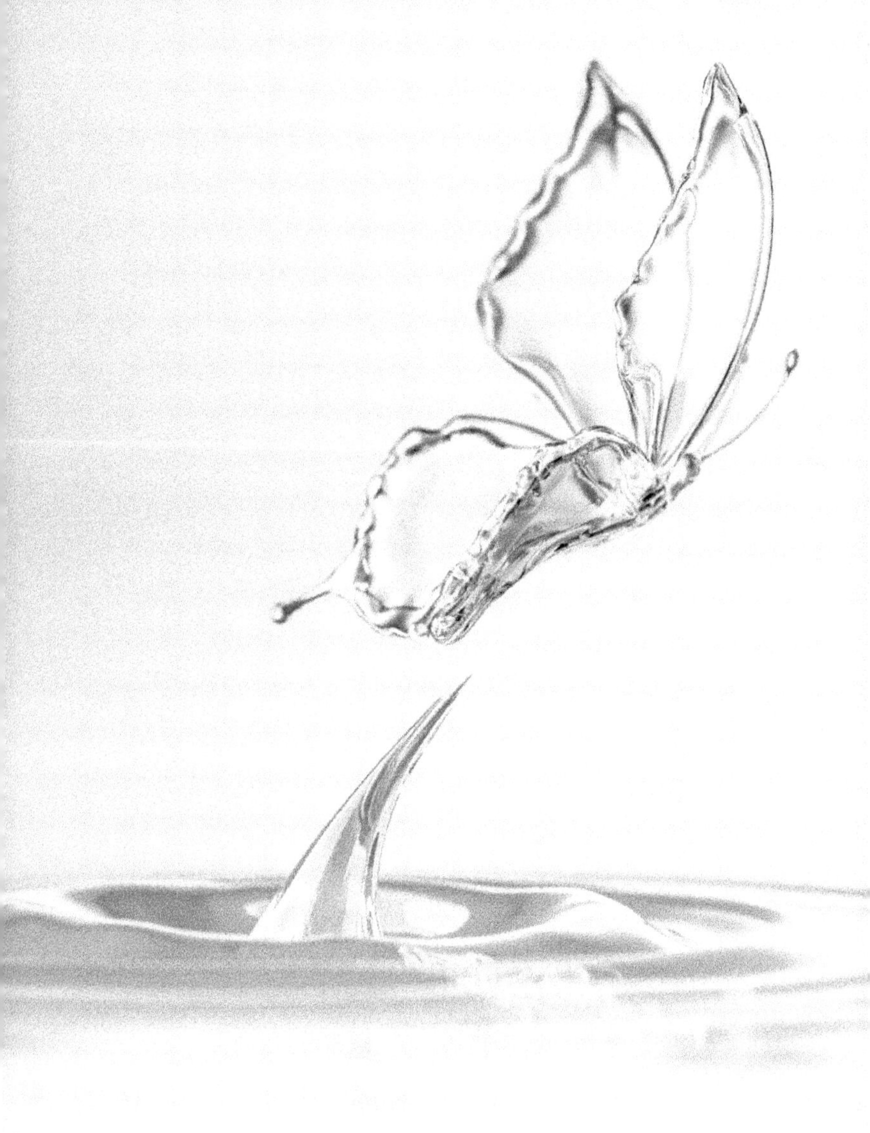

6

STRESS – THE SILENT KILLER THAT NEVER SHOWS UP ON A DEATH CERTIFICATE

Now let's take a look at the third piece of the weight gain and illness contributing trifecta: uncontrolled eating to obesity, sugar, and ***stress***.

There are three types of stress: good, bad, and ugly. In other words, creative or motivating stress, acute stress, and chronic stress. In a nutshell, creative or motivating stress can be something like buying a house, a car, getting married, etcetera. Acute stress is when you almost rear-end a car that slams on its breaks in front of you or you drop your cell phone in the lake. They have a beginning and an end. A release of stress hormones – adrenalin and cortisol among others – is immediately discharged from your adrenal glands alerting your body to fight, run, freeze, or react quickly. The third type of stress, the most dangerous, is chronic stress. That is the one we will focus on here to help you understand what it is doing to your health. The good news is you will also learn four techniques that will interrupt the stress hormones and give you relief in as little as sixty seconds. So read on.

What actually is chronic stress? Chronic stress is a continual emission of stress hormones, usually on a daily basis, that really doesn't stop. Examples of this could be an unhappy marriage, poverty, racism, a job you hate going to, COVID-19, or death of a loved one. I'm sure you can come up with some of your own, possibly something you yourself are experiencing right now. This creates what I call a drippy tap of stress hormones. They don't turn off. It's like an IV of stress hormones continually dripping into your bloodstream. This affects your sleep, your immune system, other hormones, and will absolutely stop your body from using fat for energy because your body does not know if you are running from a tiger, searching for food, or traveling across the planes. Your body still lives in the caveman era of survival and that is all it understands. So, your body thinks, "I must preserve this energy I have saved for my precious human in case we have a long wait for more food." Or, "I don't know how long we will be running from this tiger so my human will need this energy eventually." Your body will use your muscle instead of your fat if these hormones are not interrupted and in the absence of protein consumption. Thus, stress prevents weight loss. The other side-effect of untreated stress is immune system lowering. Continual stress creates a very destructive effect on your immune system thus exposing you to other diseases, allergies, stomach issues, bowel issues, hair loss, irrational behavior, skin issues, and more. Anxiety, depression, and weight gain are, therefore, all side-effects of untreated stress. In my years as a hypnotherapist, I have seen many of these ailments dissolved simply by teaching my clients how to use self-hypnosis to relax and miraculously heal. Try one or all of the following techniques to stop that drippy tap of stress hormones for yourself.

Stress is energy. Not the kind we really want all the time, but still energy. Energy has direction and movement. Everything is energy including stress and has a vibration or direction of energy. This practice will enable you to determine the direction your stress energy is moving, how to slow it down, and how to reverse it to a good, peaceful, calming feeling instead.

Practice

- First, become aware that you are feeling stress. Actually, tune in to your body because we all know we feel stress in our bodies somewhere. Mine seems to be in my solar plexus and heart area. Simply close your eyes and keep them closed when you start to feel the tension of stress and locate where in your body it is currently located. It can be anywhere. Some of my clients have felt it in their shoulders, arms, and foreheads. Your first impression of where it is located is exactly right.
- Take in a very deep breath. Keeping your eyes closed, tune into where you are feeling the stress in your body.
- Give it a rating of one to ten, one being very low and ten being "I want to run out of the room." Again, your first impression is exactly right.
- Now, using your powerful mind, I want you to actually take it slightly higher. Yes, I said higher, make it worse. If your shoulders are tense, tighten them a little

more. If your stomach feels uncomfortable make it a little more uncomfortable. This is how powerful your mind is. This also lets your mind know that you are in control and that you can lessen the stress too!

- Now use your dominant hand to indicate the direction the stress is moving as you increase it. For me, it is in a spiral. Some say moving out the top of their head, others left to right. Whatever it is, it is exactly right for you.
- Take a deep breath and continue taking deep breaths. Now reverse the direction of your hand with the intention of lowering the number you chose when you began. If the stress is moving out of the top of your head begin to move your hand down and around, down and around. For me, I reverse the spiral. Continue taking deep breaths and moving the direction of the energy in the opposite direction of when you began. In just a few moments the stress will begin to dissolve.

Congratulations, you just controlled your stress. Keep going until you feel the stress is at a level that it is no longer affecting you.

The vagus nerve runs from the brain through the face and thorax to the abdomen and interfaces with the parasympathetic control of the heart, lungs, and digestive tract.

> *"The vagal response reduces stress. It reduces our heart rate and blood pressure. It changes the function of certain parts of the brain, stimulates digestion, all those things that happen when we are relaxed."*
>
> — DR. MLADEN GOLUBIC, MD,
> MEDICAL DIRECTOR OF THE
> CLEVELAND CLINIC

Training your vagal (vagus) tone is a simple and easily practiced tool.

- Find a safe place where you can simply close your eyes. Standing or sitting works.
- Close your eyes and gaze into the space behind your eyes and let your eyelids grow heavy, heavier, very heavy.
- Drop your tongue into the bottom of your

mouth. Allow it to relax all the way to the back of your throat.

- Now take a deep diaphragm breath into and expanding your stomach.
- Exhale long, releasing all of the air, and at the same time drop your shoulders.
- Eight breaths should do it.

The more you practice this, the more automatic it becomes. Your body will naturally want to do this with time and continued practice because it feels so good and dissolves the stress hormones.

As it so happens, *stress* and *anxiety* also cause our brains to get hotter. Due to the release of stress hormones and the tightening of muscles when stress is present, your brain gets hotter. Ever heard of the saying, "Keep a cool head?" A yawn can help you achieve that.

Yawning is that ultimate stress and focus hack. Yawning clears way the fogginess of sleep and increases cerebral blood flow to cool a too-hot brain. After yawning, you quickly benefit with enhanced mental efficiency and a heightened state of cognitive awareness. In fact, yawning appears to be the fastest way to lower mental stress and anxiety. Olympic athletes yawn before they race; musicians and speakers yawn before they go on stage. Yawning is the best mental and focus hack. This book was accompanied by many yawns! I know you might be saying, "But I don't feel like yawning right now." Well then pretend.

- Rate your stress one to ten as always.
- Open your mouth wide and fake a yawn.
- Chances are you will want to do it again. Perhaps even naturally this time. Maybe even stretch your arms over your head.
- Repeat at least three times and rate your stress and motivation again.

Such an easy and simple hack – who knew!

Findings indicate that music listening impacts the psychobiological stress system. Listening to music prior to a standardized stressor predominantly affected the autonomic nervous system (in terms of a faster recovery), and to a lesser degree, the endocrine and psychological stress response. These findings may help better understanding the beneficial effects of music on the human body.

I have created a free twelve-minute relaxation and hypnotic suggestion audio for you to use in gratitude for purchasing my book and learning from these wonderful practices. It can be found at PamLeno.com. When you reach my website, a drop-down will appear asking if you would like to receive the recording. Simply by entering your email address, the download will automatically appear in your email inbox. You can download it to any device you would like! Enjoy.

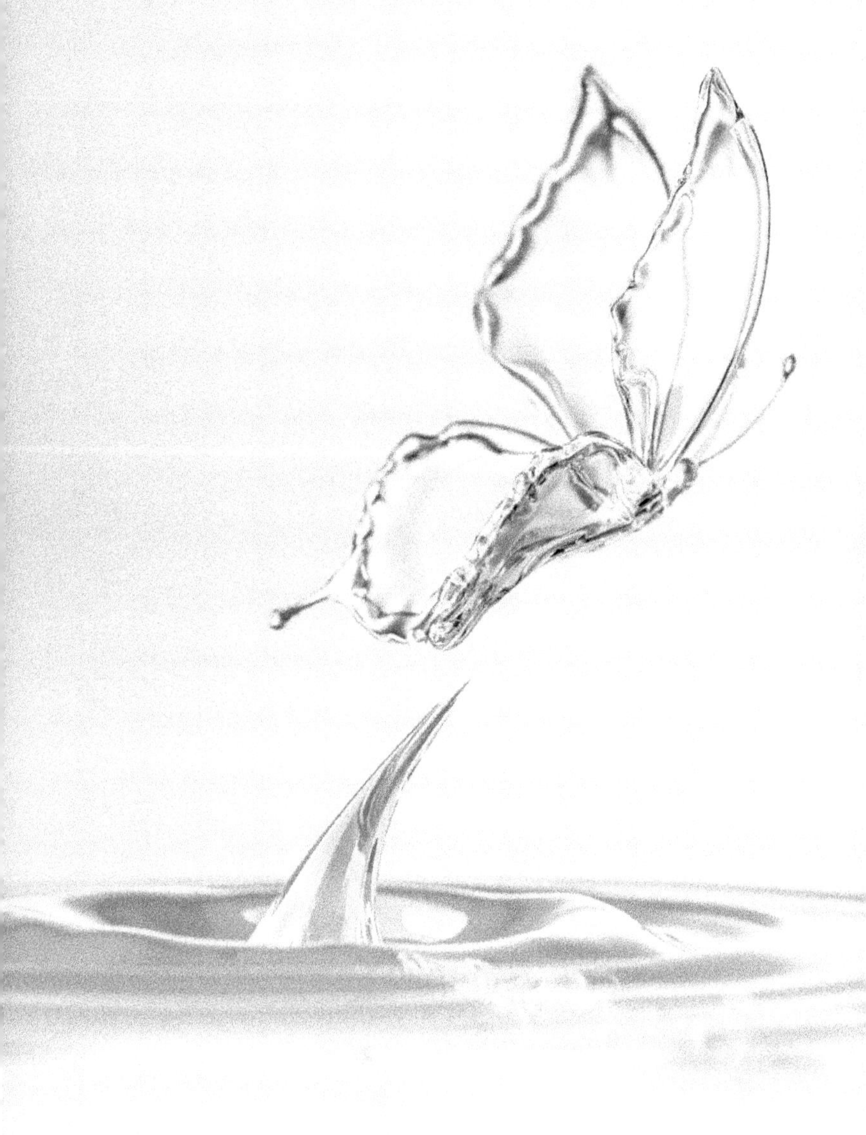

7

GUT, HEART, AND BRAIN – HEALTH FROM THE INSIDE OUT

There is a strong correlation between your heart, brain, and gut. They communicate through a series of electrical currents that create communication and if one of these systems is offline, it is like a circuit breaker in your electrical panel is off and the other two struggle to work correctly. My goal for you is to feel good and to lose weight. To have the energy and motivation to change your lifestyle and really like who you are. If your gut is not functioning well and your brain is foggy due to poor eating habits, it is very hard to hear your inner healer which is your heart. In this chapter, we are going to look at how these three areas of your body are so important and teach you a technique to bring them into coherence.

Remember the vagus nerve we discussed in Chapter 6? This nerve plays an important role in the communication of your gut, brain, and heart.

GUT

Let's start with the gut. Not only does the gut "talk" to the brain chemically, but it also sends electric signals via the vagus nerve. The vagus nerve relays information and status of internal organs like gut and heart to the brain and vice versa. It is the communication highway for all internal organs. Most of the gut neurons are used in the daily grind of digestion. Gut systems are an extremely complex chemical processing machine which breaks down the food, absorbs nutrients, and moves the waste down to expel it. Thus, the autonomous nervous system of the gut allows it to work independently of the brain.

However, the gut is mostly sending information to the brain and not the other way around. The reverse interaction from the brain to the gut is when we get hunger pangs, and the brain tells the body to get food or when something goes wrong in the gut like acid reflux, digestive issues, constipation, diarrhea, or bloating from the consumption of unhealthy foods. Recent scientific evidence also suggests that a big part of our emotions is probably influenced by the chemicals and nerves in the gut. For example, 95 percent of the body's serotonin is found in the gut. Serotonin is an important neurotransmitter which is a well-known contributor toward feelings of well-being – the happiness hormone. So, the gut plays an important role in our physical health as well as our mental health, as you can see. If your gut is not in harmony, you will not feel good.

Keeping your gut flora healthy by eating fresh vegetables, eating lean proteins, drinking lots of water, and keeping carbohydrates (especially yeast-refined foods and white flour) at a minimum result in a healthier gut. Eating raw and fermented vegetables provides fiber and much needed probiotics to keep your gut healthy. Vegetables also make you feel full and satisfied which helps with weight loss. A diet that is mainly plant-based with some healthy, lean protein for muscle support, occasional fruits, nuts, seeds, and whole grains really makes your tummy and body happy.

Jolyn came to me with such a bad acid reflux (heart burn) issue that she was on a prescription medication that had to be taken daily just for her to feel okay. She was very overweight, and her diet consisted of fast food, cereal, more fast food. The problem was that her gut was so unbalanced that she was presenting too much stomach acid in response to what she was eating and it hurt. We discussed her diet and changed what she was eating to more vegetables and cleaner protein plus increased her water intake. She began to practice the stress reduction techniques I taught her. Was it easy? Not at first. She put the effort in and by week four we were able to remove the prescription medications. Interestingly enough, taste buds change when diet is changed especially with the decrease or removal of sugar. Jolyn reported that she didn't really like vegetables at first however as her gut healed and she continued to consume fresh lovely vegetables she actually began to like them. She experimented with new ways of preparation and as her gut healed, her weight went down, too. Today she is still medication-free and has lost 65 pounds. Was it worth the effort? What do you think?

The heart is one of the most important organs of the human body. Life starts when the heart starts beating and ends when it stops. There are nearly 2 billion muscle cells and 40,000 neurons in the heart. The heart-mind interaction takes place both by electrical signals via the vagus nerve and the spinal cord nerves and through body chemicals.

Recent studies have shown that heart sends signals to the brain and are not only understood by it but are also obeyed. Scientists have discovered neural pathways and mechanisms whereby input from heart to brain inhibits or facilitates the brain's electrical activity. – just like the gut. Thus, both gut and heart help the overall thought process and foster wellbeing.

Besides the electrical signaling, the heart is also an endocrine gland realizing peptides which help in blood pressure modulation and improving the functioning of kidneys. These peptides also stimulate the pituitary gland thereby helping it to release hormones like oxytocin commonly referred to as the "love" or "bonding" hormone. Oxytocin also helps with increasing the wellbeing of a person. This could be the basis of saying that happy feelings emanate from the heart.

The speed of the heartbeat changes depending upon our emotions. For example, when we are aroused either by passion or anger, then the heart speeds up and in more quiet times or self-hypnosis, it slows down. That is why the stress reduction techniques in Chapter 6 work so well – they are forming a communication circuit through breath and the vagus nerve to create the beneficial effect and coherence of the gut, brain, and heart!

Here is an interesting fact to consider about the heart. Did you know that the heart is the only organ that can live outside of the body for a period of time?

Also, the heart has memory. Some studies have been done with patients that received heart transplants from donors. People that received the heart have begun to desire foods that they never ate in the past – for instance, spicy foods. When they meet the family of the donor, the family reported how much the donor loved spicy food! Another fascinating example is of a young girl receiving a heart transplant and after a period of time she began having nightmares about a man trying to kill her. The mother became concerned and spoke with the child's doctor. Upon further research, the donor of the heart had actually been murdered! Being wise and not ignoring what was going on, the police were contacted, and the child was able to identify the murderer and he was arrested! So, feelings, intuition, and love are all emitting from your heart.

I work with the education and teachings from an institute in California called the HeartMath Institute™ (HeartMath.com).

HeartMath™ has developed a research-based system of scientifically validated techniques, tools, and technology to increase emotional and mental self-regulation. The tools can help us gain greater self-regulation and a new perspective. Most of the HeartMath™ techniques include an intentional shift to a positive emotional state to help gain coherence. The Heart-Focused Breathing Technique™ is a powerful tool to practice and gain an ability to neutralize emotions such as anxiety and anger.

The Heart-Focused Breathing Technique™ is an easy-to-use, energy-saving, self-regulation strategy. It is designed to reduce the intensity of a stress reaction and to establish a calm, but alert state. The presence of stress hormones slows the ability of the body to use fat for energy. When you can gain control of stress hormones simply by using the techniques presented in this book you increase the chances of a more peaceful life and slimmer body. The technique allows you to take a time-out where you can step back and neutralize your depleting emotions. We can benefit from conscious breathing, if we use it to help us shift into and sustain a more balanced state. Breathing is only the start of what is known as a coherence-building process.

In addition, the Heart-Focused Breathing™ helps

reduce the impact of stress on your mind and body. It helps us reduce the energy drain in order to feel a bit more renewed. By going to a neutral state, it helps us to detach from our emotionally charged feelings and racing mind. By practicing this technique, it gives us an opportunity to pause our thoughts and feelings long enough to consider the possible options and consequences.

Step One: Focus your attention on the area of your heart. Imagine your breath is flowing in and out of your heart or chest area. Breathe a little deeper and slower than usual.

- Try and inhale for a count of five, and exhale for a count of five
- Once you have become familiar with this step, all you need to remember is the quick step to neutralize stress

Step Two: Bring in a thought of someone, something, or some place you love. Keep your mental picture on whatever it is and *feel* the love that you are emotionally experiencing.

Step Three: Notice how you feel – peaceful, calm, or centered.

Suggestions for when to practice the Heart-Focused Breathing Technique™:

1. Stop the impact of stress on your body instead of heading for the fridge.
2. Help neutralize emotional reactions in the moment – like eating when you are really not hungry.
3. Eliminate the energy drain, like when you are struggling to focus.
4. Remove the drama or significance of a situations, such as coworkers gossip.
5. Reenergize and open your creative intuition. Need a creative idea?
6. Problem-solve.

Now you have some tools for your toolbox! Tools only work if you pick them up and use them. Practice one or two of these until you have them mastered. Then add another one and you now have a foolproof-coherence method between gut, heart, and mind (brain). In the next chapter, we will focus our attention more to the brain and how powerful our thoughts are. I will also teach you to harness this power and use it to your advantage on your weight-loss journey.

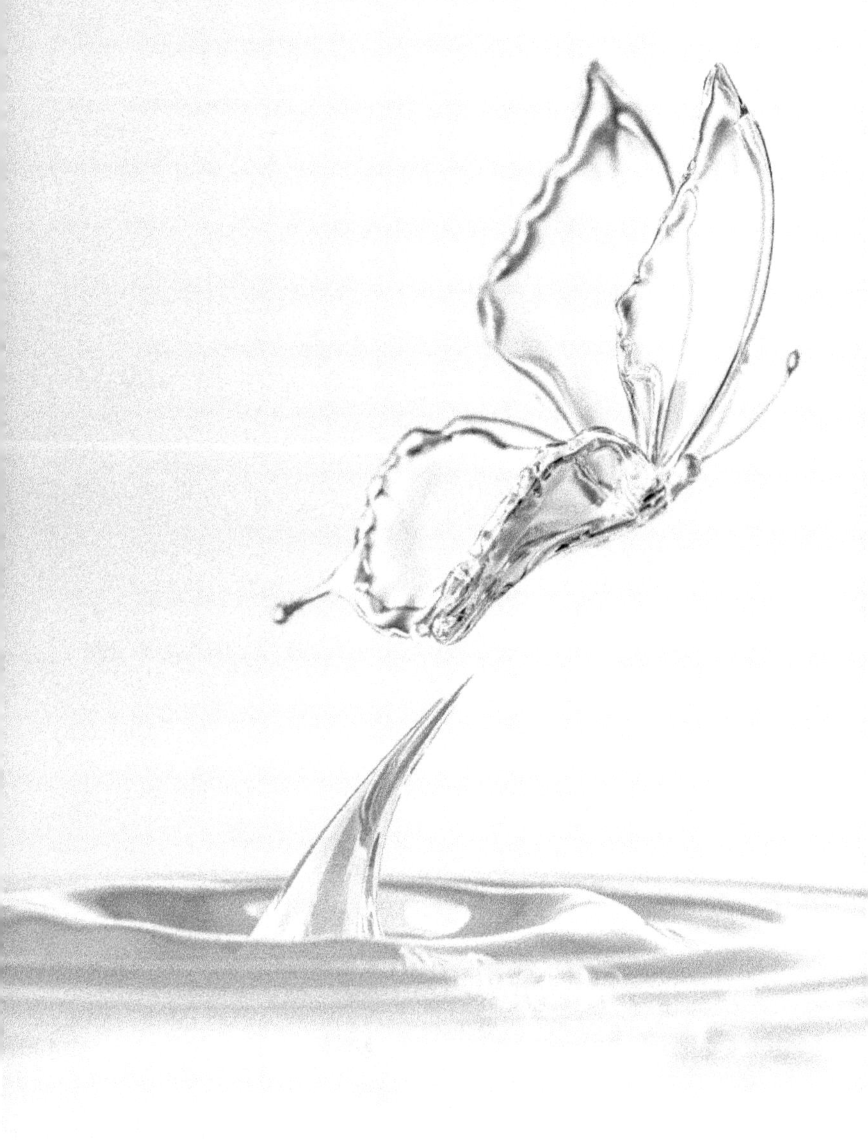

8

TOSS THE THOUGHT – RETRAIN YOUR THOUGHTS TO SUPPORT YOUR SUCCESS

As Dr. Wayne Dyer, internationally renowned author and speaker, states, "Your thoughts become things." This is more true than most people give it. Here is an example for you to try.

Close your eyes for a moment and take a deep breath.

Next, I want you to think about the tips of your fingers tingling. Yes, tingling, tingling, tingling. Maybe you even feel it moving up into your fingers. The tingling sensation is becoming stronger.

I can almost guarantee that you actually felt your fingers tingling! Simply by putting that focused thought into your mind, your body reacted.

Let's try another one. Close your eyes and

imagine a big juicy lemon. Now pretend to take a big bite! What happened to your mouth? Pucker? Saliva production? Yes, your thoughts produce things, feelings, emotions.

So, if you are thinking poorly about yourself, not liking what you see in the mirror, demeaning yourself because of how your clothes fit, comparing yourself to other thinner people – these thoughts are creating a reaction in your body! These thoughts do not feel good. They destroy cells and slow down your immune system. They affect your nervous system. There is a hormonal reaction as well. Adrenalin and cortisol are released. These are stress hormones. These negative thoughts actually carry an energy that your body responds to without you even realizing it except that you feel bad and then worse. Then your brain wants comfort, so what do you do? Eat. Because at this point your brain and body are just looking for some way to feel better based on how horrible your thoughts are making them feel. Remember, you were taught that soothing comes from putting something in your mouth from the time you entered this world. Thus, the eat-feel-bad-eat cycle begins.

My plan for you is to create optional feel-good processes to turn to instead of food. In Chapter 9, you will learn an amazing brain hack called "Toss the Thought" that actually reverses and reframes these thoughts to positive, self-affirming feel-good thoughts that actually support your immune system, your cells, and your self-control.

YOUR INNER FOUR-YEAR-OLD

Your reptilian brain, the first part of our brains to develop, is kind of like a four-year-old. You see that nicely packed chocolate cake at the store. You know it will not support your healthy lifestyle or weight loss. However, your reptilian brain (your inner four-year-old) is throwing a fit on the grocery store floor saying it wants it. Maybe it's that bag of Doritos or the tub of ice cream. Your inner four-year-old will argue with you, cry, whine, and eventually throw itself on the floor in a fit. You can try to negotiate, control your inner four-year-old, talk some sense into her, hold her, or…now this sounds crazy; take a deep breath and walk away. Yes, it can be a scary thing to do. Nevertheless, eventually the inner four-year-old will stop the fit and come find you. She did not get what she wanted but now no one is paying attention to her. That is how I want you to think about those cravings, negative thoughts or thoughts about eating the foods that will not support your goals. Walk away. Find a more satisfying thing to do like call a friend, paint, go for a walk, sing, create something, watch funny videos; whatever it is, exit the area of your inner four-year-old throwing a tantrum. It will get easier and easier. Remember you are the adult here.

POSITIVE THINKING

Yes, you have control of your thinking, but no one has taught you how to at this point. I will teach you the practices to use as tools. You cannot fix a leaky faucet without first picking up the tools. That is a must for this to work here. Using the tools you will learn in Chapters 6 and 9, you can regain control of your negative thoughts and convert them to positive, life-affirming thoughts, feelings, and results. That happens easily once you employ your awareness and practice.

Let's talk about how your body responds to positive thoughts.

A loving, caring thought affects your hormones. Like, "I am doing so well! This is really working and I feel great!" Or, "I feel so much better eating the fresh vegetables that I know are so good for me." Just as negative thinking incites the production of adrenalin and cortisol, affirmative thoughts cause the release of dopamine, the neurotransmitter for the brain's reward system; serotonin which regulates mood, sleep, appetite, digestion, learning, and memory; oxytocin, the love hormone; and endorphins which are your natural pain reliever. So, it is easy to see that if these hormones are not produced your body, mind, and soul are not in alignment and the result is eat feel-bad-eat-feel-bad cycle.

TOSS THE THOUGHT

This technique is a bit of a brain hack or trick to allow you to take back control of negative self-destructive talk. We all have thoughts about ourselves that steal our good feelings about ourselves and set us up for remorse, guilt, shame, etcetera. This technique will teach you how to promptly and efficiently reframe those thoughts to positive, energizing, healing thoughts that will lead you to fulfillment, self-satisfaction, and joy!

If I am holding my right hand out on the right side of my body, then the left side of my brain is engaged and active. However, if I move my right hand across the midline of my body to the left side of my body, then the right side of my brain is engaged. So even though it is still my right hand that is now on the left side of my body, my brain has flipped sides.

Here is how you can use this to your benefit.

First, you must be aware of your thoughts and if they feel good or not. It is a physical response as mentioned above.

Let's say you have a self-limiting thought like, "I'm not good enough," "I am fat," "I can't do this," etcetera. Is that what you want? If the answer is no, then imagine that the thought actually has a physical presence because really it kind of does as it is affecting your body. Literally, grab the thought in your hand; let's say you use your right hand and toss it across your body to the left side of your body and throw it away. Then, return the hand to the right side of your body and open it face up and say, "What I really want is…" Then restate the thought to something like, "To be healthy, feel good about myself, be successful and I want to feel happy, grateful, energetic etcetera." This will change the cellular vibration and you will begin to feel better immediately. The more you practice this the easier and automatic it will become, and you literally can begin to reframe your life by what you are thinking. Here is the link to a YouTube video I made to show you how to do this: https://www.youtube.com/watch?v=mtkSTB0eFyQ. As you practice this, you will actually feel the physical effects of changing your thought. This truly can change your life. I use it daily. This is a conscious technique and first you must be aware of where your thoughts are going. Practice is key.

In the next chapter, we will begin to learn and practice the superpower of self-hypnosis. Self-hypnosis is like a power tool for your toolbox. It is what plugs into the outlet, the source of all power and success – your Higher Power.

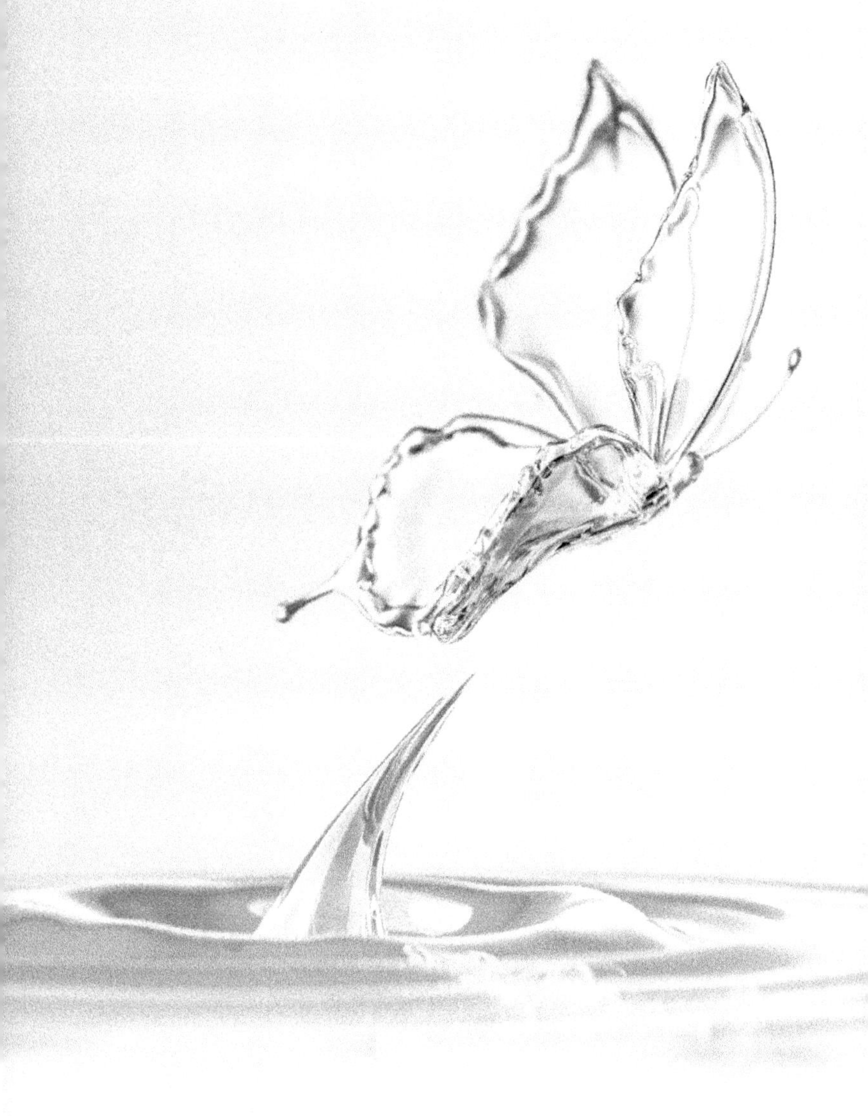

9

SELF-HYPNOSIS AND DECLARATIONS – THE SOULUTION

Hypnosis is focused attention. You have actually been in hypnosis many times. For example, do you remember the first time you drove a car? You were very focused. You thought of nothing else and paid attention to every turn, braking, signaling, etcetera. Now, however, you can drive from point A to point B and not remember what you passed on the way! In most cases, your mind is somewhere else completely. This is a form of self-hypnosis. Your subconscious mind is driving the car while your conscious mind is thinking of something else completely.

Let's look at the three minds that you have – the conscious mind, the subconscious mind, and the unconscious mind. These three minds are kind of like a computer. The conscious mind is the monitor or screen. It is in the moment; someone must touch keys or something to make any changes to the screen. Only small amounts of information can be observed at any one period. Your subconscious mind is like the hard drive of your computer. Every single bit of information that has ever taken place from the time you left the womb is stored there. The problem with that is some of the files may have a virus or perhaps outdated and untrue information that is somehow still affecting the other files on the hard drive. The unconscious mind is like the power cord that plugs into the wall and without you knowing it operates the complete system. Without this power cord, you would not be able to operate. Hypnosis works at the subconscious or hard drive level. In hypnosis, we can access the files that are no longer serving us, either delete them or change them to actually assist in changing from the inside out.

My method of self-hypnosis is the connection with your Higher Power, whatever you conceptualize that to be. This is a spiritual practice not to be confused with religion. For this method, it is important for your connection to whatever you consider your Higher Power to be a loving and trusting relationship. It is welcoming of this Higher Power to be a part of this process. Inviting It to be your friend, your companion, someone you can trust in and feel like It has your back, something you can lean on, that provides relief and hope. It helps in situations when you feel like you can't do it on your own. It intuitively reminds you that you are a powerful being. It is your bestie! This is the power cord for your computer and all the minds.

This Power is greater than any willpower you try. It's better that any therapist or magic pill. This Power is truly your Savior on your weight loss or any other journey. When you establish a relationship with It, things change. When you communicate with It daily, life gets better. When you trust It and stay plugged in things go much more smoothly. The problem is our conscious mind, our ego, can get in the way. We try to do it by ourselves. Pushing ourselves forward with our free will and willpower and forgetting to ask for the help we need for that which literally created us. We all have freewill. That is our option to choose for ourselves. Sometimes we choose what is best for us and sometimes we don't. The great thing about plugging into your Higher Power is that you don't have to do it by yourself. This Power is the generator of your life. Why not attach your cords and live from a space of peace?

Meaning of Declaration: The Formal Announcement of the Beginning of a State or Condition

You are formally announcing that you are ready – really ready – to make the changes you wish to achieve.

You are declaring your connection and faith in your Higher Power or Source

Declarations are words that invite and invoke your Higher Power to be a participant in this journey of weight loss and a healthier, happier lifestyle.

You will learn how to use them to induce a level of self-hypnosis. This is a relaxed state of mind and body that you will be able to achieve simply by following the technique and recording access that will be provided at the end of this chapter

They can be used as affirmations daily with your eyes open to stay plugged in.

They can be used as meditation or prayer.

With your words, you will be declaring what you are saying to be your truth, exactly what you really want in your life. You will be inviting your Higher Power to assist in the process of your success. You surrender your problem and allow your Higher Power to take it from you, to release you from its grips, to lighten your load, and to provide relief, hope, healing and joy!

DECLARATIONS

Here is your First Declaration

Part One: (name of your Higher Power) I believe in Your power to assist and support my success.

Part Two: To provide an inner strength that I know I cannot do alone. Thank You.

Second Declaration

Part One: I gratefully accept Your will in my life.

Part Two: And I willingly release my unwanted extra weight to You.

Part Three: Take this burden from me so I may feel joy, love, and peace. Thank You.

Third Declaration

Part One: I trust You (name your Higher Power) to give me the strength.

Part Two: courage, faith, and clarity

Part Three: I need to achieve the health I desire now always and forever.

Practice

These declarations are powerful. As you practice daily, at least two times for no longer than twenty minutes and upon going to sleep at night, these begin to create new neurological connections in your brain – in other words, *new habits*! Our goal is to have these become an automated response for you upon waking, during the day and going to sleep at night – an automated response to stress, the desire to eat when you are not hungry, anxiety – whatever is causing you to turn to food for comfort.

You are inviting your Higher Power to be a participant in your success! There is level of faith here. It is the same kind of faith you have in gravity. You can't see gravity or know how it really works. However, you don't doubt it. You expect it to keep you on the earth as well as your car, furniture, or house for that matter. That is the kind of faith at work here. It requires a certain level of belief that defies our human nature of seeing everything in our current environments. It is a belief that what you desire is completely possible. It is a faith that is like a river running to the sea. It does not doubt that it will reach the sea regardless of the rocks, cliffs, or other obstacles. The faith of the acorn falling from the tree has that it will eventually grow into a tree, too. The faith of the seed in the ground to grow into a plant. Positive energy – that is the faith I am asking you to bring to these declarations and techniques. If you can do that, you will get results. Believe it is possible.

Try it out and just see what you experience in your very first time. My dream for you is that you will experience a new sense of relief, hope, and lightness

HOW TO INDUCE SELF-HYPNOSIS

As promised, here is how to begin the practice of self-hypnosis. Read the directions first and then practice each bullet point with eyes open before you move to eyes closed.

Find a safe place where you will not be disturbed and can safely close your eyes for the intended duration of your practice.

- Look up at the ceiling and take a deep breath.
- Continue to stare at the ceiling and breathing deeply until your eyes want to close.
- Now gaze into the space behind your closed eyes and let your eyelids grow heavy, heavy, heavy.
- Allow your tongue to drop into the bottom of your mouth and relax all the way to the back of your throat.
- Use your vagus nerve relaxation technique

by taking in another deep breath and on the exhale, allow your shoulders to drop and your ribcage to relax and drop toward your hips.

- Let that relaxation move down your body – abdomen, hips, thighs, knees, calves, tops of feet bottom of feet – all the way to the tips of your toes.
- Take in another deep breath extending your stomach out (diaphragm breathing). Hold your breath to the count of five.
- Exhale every single ounce of air you can and allow your body to sink into the chair.
- As you breathe normally visualize a perfect scene from nature. Place yourself in the scene. Wherever you wish to go is perfect.
- Feel the air, hear the sounds, notice what is around you. Truly allow yourself to feel the elements of where you are.
- Notice how relaxed your mind and body are.
- Now is the time to practice the declarations in your own mind.
- Say the declaration to yourself.
- Wait for whatever follows, a thought,

picture, memory, color. Whatever it is, it is perfect. Then return to the declaration. Do not judge or ask yourself, "Am I doing this right?" You are allowing your subconscious mind to focus and relax, focus and relax. Retraining your own brain!

PRACTICE SCHEDULE

Daily practice is recommended.

This practice does take commitment. I promise you the results are worth it. Think of something that you have done that you are really proud of. Did it happen overnight? Probably not. You worked at it. Practiced. Stuck with it. And – success! The same applies here. Don't rush it. If you want to remain in one declaration for more than a week, great! If you want to stay with Part One or Part Two longer, great! If you want to jump ahead earlier than weekly, great! Make it your practice. You are creating within you and your connection with your Power Source. This is a process. Remember that Rome was not built in a day. Be patient with yourself and enjoy!

Week One: Begin with just the first declaration, part one, and practice two to three times a day for ten to twenty minutes with eyes closed for one week. Remember you can use these as affirmations throughout the day and I highly recommend it. I love using them when I am hiking in nature.

Week Two: Add part two of declaration one. Feel free to open your eyes to remember the words. When I started, I had to have them on paper or my phone next to me to remember. I would peak at them and close my eyes and repeat until I had them memorized.

Week Three: Add part one of declaration two and split the intended practice time into halves. For instance, practice declaration one in full for ten minutes and part one of declaration two for ten minutes. Feel free to have them next to you and peek at them as needed. It will not change the outcome.

Week Four: Add part two of declaration two and again split intended practice time between declaration one full and parts one and two of declaration two.

Week Five: Add part three of declaration three and again split intended practice time between declaration one in full and now declaration two in full.

Week Six: Add part one of declaration three. Split intended practice time between declarations one and two in full and part one of declaration three. Be gentle with yourself and do not be frustrated if you cannot remember all the words or forget a few right away. You will get to the point of an automated response.

Week Seven: Add part two of declaration three. Now split time equally with the three declarations you have.

Week Eight: Add part three of declaration three. Congratulations you have them all!

There are more declarations to move into and I will tell you how to get them at the end of this book. This practice changed my life. I have a completely different relationship with my Higher Power now and love the response It has had on the inspiration, peace, joy, and delight I have in my life now. Of course, I have down days; we all do. I just choose to lift myself with the assistance of my Higher Power and not stay there too long.

NEW FEELINGS TO EXPECT

Gina was sitting at her office desk when a coworker came by and started telling her about a situation they had been working on together and attempted to undermine a decision Gina had already made as a manager concerning the situation. In the past, Gina would get angry, say something she regretted, and let it stress her out for the rest of the day, maybe the week. Then she'd go home and eat everything she could see to try to make herself feel better!

Interestingly, this time around, she noticed that she remained calm and responded in a manner that showed compassion for the co-worker's actions. Gina was able to easily respond in a manner of understanding. She noticed she didn't even think about it on the way home. Actually, she felt great upon arrival and ate a healthy meal and relaxed for the evening. Now that's measurable.

The changes you will experience are not lightning bolt magical. You will notice subtle changes. You may find yourself responding to situations where in the past you would have reacted, gotten upset, or tried eating to soothe the uncomfortableness of emotions. Now you realize that all emotions are great. They are trying to tell you something and believe me *it is not to eat* to make them go away! To further your understanding of your emotions and what they are trying to tell you I highly recommend Cal Banyan's book *The Secret Language of Feelings*. Cal has been a great influence in my life with his work both in 5-PATH hypnotherapy and 7th Path self-hypnosis. Much of what I am writing about here has evolved from his teaching.

New feelings of calmness, peace, and a wonderful self-control will begin to make themselves known as you trust your Higher Power, practice the declarations, and believe in your Higher Power and yourself. As we reduce the stress hormones with the techniques in Chapter 6 and begin this connection with your Higher Power, inevitably your body and mind can return to homeostasis. Balance. Love. Peace. Hormonal balance can be restored. Isn't that nice?

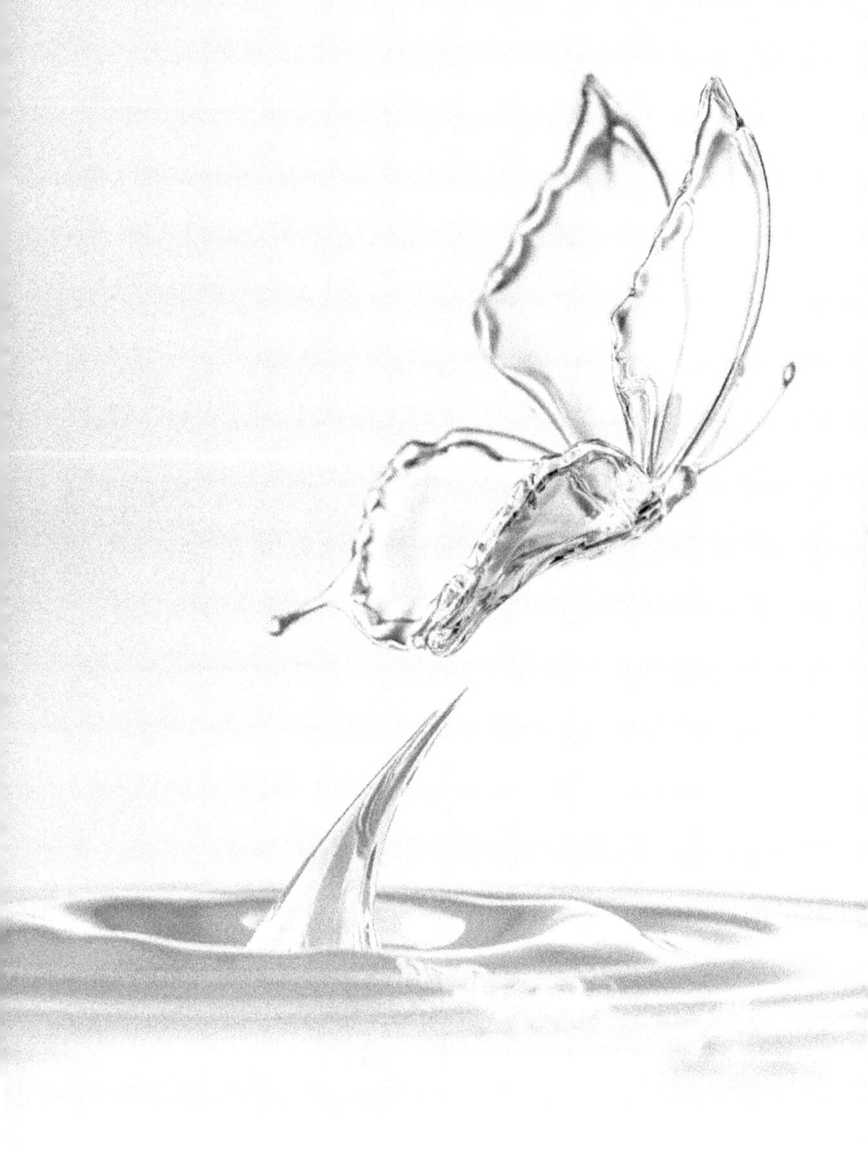

10

A GUIDED FUTURE PROGRESSION SELF-HYPNOSIS TECHNIQUE

It has been long known that visualization is a key factor in how your life is going. An example is a vacation. You first decide where you want to go. You look at brochures, search the internet, and begin to form a picture or visualization of where you want to go. Next, you decide when, how to get there, rental cars, where you are staying, and what you will do when you are there. Basically, you begin with the end in mind and then plan backward. You get excited, buy clothes, prepare as if it has already happened. The same philosophy applies to your life, but you rarely think of it that way. Some of the most successful people I know visualize on a daily basis. They consider how they want their lives to be, how they want to feel, what their businesses are doing, who they are dating, etcetera. They actually close their eyes, see themselves already in the place they want to get to and how they want to feel. This is the law of attraction. I did it with my home on a lake. It was, frankly, financially out of my reach based on where I was at the moment, but I drove there often, saw myself entering the house, feeling the peace and contentment of being there. Guess where I live now! Yep! On that lake, in that house I dreamed of. I have done the same with dream car purchases, life partners, and my business, so I know for a fact that this works! Follow the directions next; you can also listen to a guided recording at Weight-LossHypnosisBook.com. Only special people who have purchased and read this book have access so congratulations! You are one of my special people! I love and appreciate you!

First, find a safe comfortable place to relax and close your eyes where you will not be disturbed.

Close your eyes and follow the self-hypnosis directions in Chapter 9. Since we are talking about weight loss in this book, let's focus on that however this technique can be used for any area of your life you wish to improve.

Next, visualize yourself on a path somewhere

that you can imagine you would enjoy a walk. This is the pathway to success, feeling great, a slimmer, healthier you. Eating healthy nutritious foods and avoiding the foods you know are not good for you based on what you learned in the first chapters of this book. Now in your mind's eye, imagine you are seeing yourself on a movie or TV screen one year into practicing healthy eating habits, moving your body with joy, however that looks to you. You have lost weight and are feeling energized, happy, healthy. On that movie screen, see a picture of yourself one year in the future. How much weight have you lost? What are you wearing? What color are the clothes you have on? Are you indoors or out? Alone or with someone? Who, if anyone, is there? Now as you see yourself healthy, happy, slimmer, notice how you feel. Lighter? More energized? Excited? Yes! You are creating these feelings mentally, physically, and emotionally. As you tune into this wonderful feeling, determine where exactly in your body are those feelings radiating from. As you pinpoint the location give it a color. Your first impression is exactly right. Now using your magical mind expand the color, make it bigger. Yes, you can; remember that your mind is very powerful. Keep expanding the color and the feeling into every cell, every hair follicle, every neuron in your brain, every blood vessel until your whole body is vibrating with this feeling. Great!

Now bringing that feeling with you and going back to your screen imagine yourself five years in the future on that screen. You have continued to eat healthy, move your body joyfully. See yourself there now! Look at how wonderful you look, feel, move. What are you wearing? What color are your clothes? Are you indoors or out? Alone or with someone? What is happening? What are you doing? Just repeat the exercise from above bringing as much detail as you can onto the screen. Now, this is you in the future. Let's call her Future Self and you are you in the past. Let me tell you about Future Self. She is you. So, everything she tells you is absolute truth. Isn't that nice!? So here is your opportunity to ask her anything you would like to know that will help you get to where she is. Take this time now just between the two of you to ask anything you would like. The immediate response from your future self can only assist you. Her answers can only give you the keys, tools, ideas that will help you get to where she is five years from now. Make this scene beautiful, full of color and vibrancy. Have a conversation with yourself and really allow the true you in your future to speak. When you feel like you have the answers you want, thank your future self for being here today. Now just imagine the two of you standing, and embracing each other, allowing a joining of the souls to occur. You may now allow that scene to fade, knowing that you have just created your future.

This is a change you have made for yourself at a subconscious level. These changes are permanent. By using the education of the first chapters of this book, practicing self-hypnosis and connecting with your Higher Power plus this future progression and visualizing yourself successful, healthy, and happy you are establishing new building blocks in your subconscious mind. Will you need to revisit these practices? Yes, often. The more you can visualize bring in the feeling and take physical steps toward your healthy, slim, happy self you can achieve. What you believe you can achieve. You can reignite your inner light and shine it for all to see.

Here is a quote from one of my favorite authors Marianne Williamson. I had the privilege of working with her in the creation of this book – an amazing author and promotor of love in our world.

> *"Our deepest fear is not that we are inadequate. Our deepest fear is that we are powerful beyond measure. It is our light, not our darkness that most frightens us. We ask ourselves, 'Who am I to be brilliant, gorgeous, talented, fabulous?' Actually, who are you not to be? You are a child of God. Your playing small does not serve the world. There is nothing enlightened about shrinking so that other people won't feel insecure around you. We are all meant to shine, as children do. We were born to make manifest the glory of God that is within us. It's not just in some of us; it's in everyone. And as we let our own light shine, we unconsciously give other people permission to do the same. As we are liberated from our own fear, our presence automatically liberates others."*
>
> — MARIANNE WILLIAMSON

Keeping this in mind and in your heart is not prideful or self-centered. Imagine yourself healthy strong and beautiful. It is your right. You were born perfect. You are completely lovable and there is nothing wrong with you. Your creator did not make a mistake when It created you. You were put on this earth to live a life of love, joy, and empowerment. It is time for you to take the steps, practice the techniques, return yourself to love. The most powerful emotion is love. The opposite of love is fear. Everything that is not love is fear. Where are you living and where do you want to go? Here is a link to your future progression audio for a guided visualization and self-hypnosis: WeightLossHypnosisBook.com

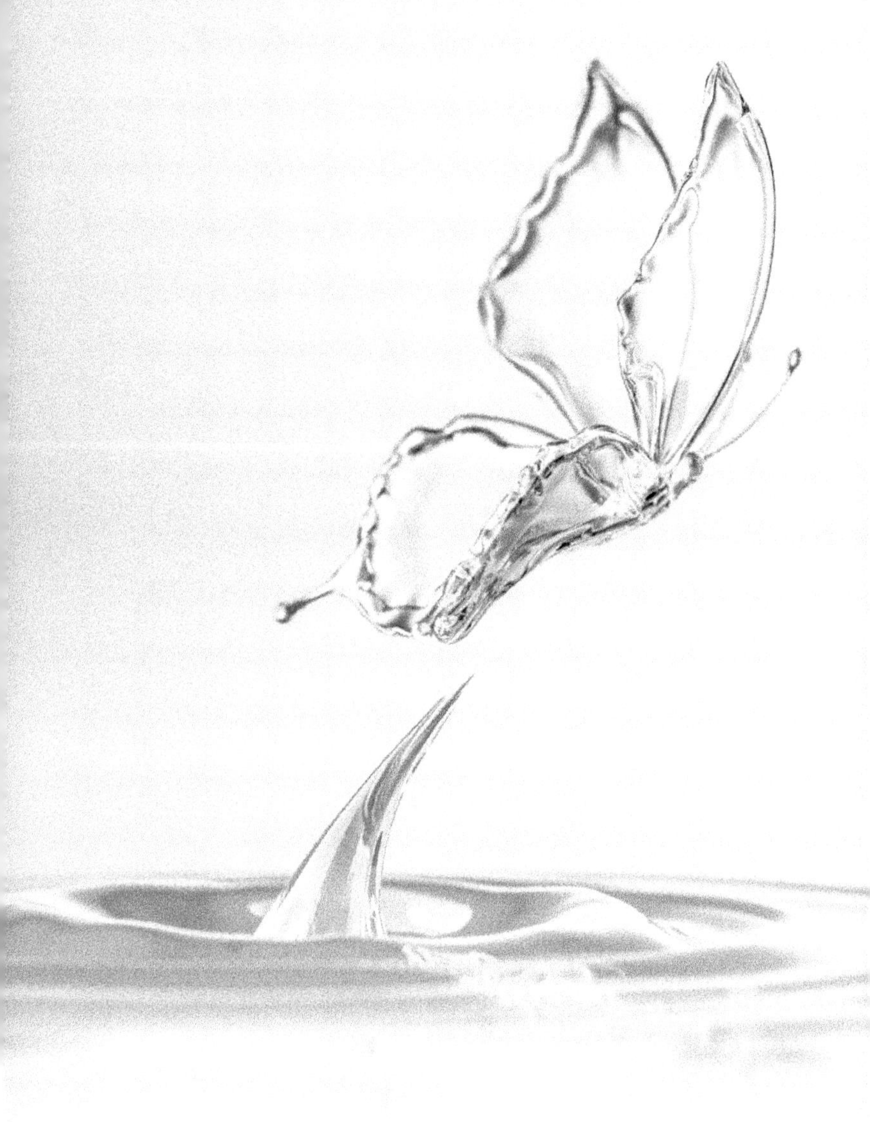

11

RESULTS YOU CAN MEASURE

Will your results be lightning-bolt fast? Probably not. This is a process that shows results over a period of time. Remember, you did not put on the extra weight overnight. It will take some effort on your part by using the information on how food affects your body and make healthier choices based on your new knowledge. Remember that one pound of fat has 3,500 calories of energy to burn. Knowing that, keep your carbohydrates and fat lower than what you are currently doing and move your body, and you *will* lose fat. Practice your self-hypnosis daily, drink water, visualize, use the stress reduction tools; all this will benefit you physically, mentally, emotionally, and spiritually.

My clients report that they "just" feel more peaceful and calmer. They notice that things that used to bother them or make them eat emotionally just don't have the same effect. Kind of like water off a duck's back. Sleep improves, which of course also reduces the stress hormones, and we now know what damage that can have on our health. You may notice that as your gut flora changes you no longer want to eat the sugary, unhealthy foods because they make you feel like crap. Your energy increases because you are getting lighter and feeling better about yourself and your body. You may find yourself smiling more – generally feeling happier for no reason in particular.

I highly recommend you track your own progress by writing down your experience. It is important to recognize your successes, whatever they are and give yourself credit for something as simple as eating a serving size of chips and not the whole bag. Hug yourself for resisting the craving for something and walking away to find something more satisfying than succumbing to your inner four-year-old's tantrum. Celebrate the success of taking a walk instead of eating the cake. Creating a healthy tasty meal is an amazing victory; take it in. And ultimately, congratulate yourself on the success of the scale showing your results.

As you gain the acknowledgment on paper, your subconscious mind begins to realize and understand that this is who you really are and support you in your progress. Especially as you begin to reframe your thoughts to those of success. As you begin to notice your negative, self-degrading thoughts write them down. Using the "Toss the Thought" method from Chapter 8, write your new self-affirming thought. Getting your cellular vibration into alignment with your positive outcomes. Here is a checklist of ten things for you to consider that will improve as you continue your practices.

1. Check on your feelings of calmness and peace. Give the feeling a rating of one to ten (one being stressed and tense, and ten being calm and at peace within). If you are feeling like a one, do one of the stress reduction techniques from Chapter 6 and increase your feelings of peace and calmness up the scale! Remember, this takes practice and effort.
2. What are you thinking right now and how are those thoughts making you feel? As

you continue to practice journaling your thinking and using the "Toss the Thought" method, you will notice those old negative thoughts dissipate. Check in.

3. Step on the scale once a week. Track your progress.
4. Journal about what has changed in your eating habits this week. List all improvements and congratulate yourself on every little win. For instance, today I ate on half of my plate and felt completely full when in the past I would have eaten everything on my plate and went back for seconds!
5. Are you moving your body with joy? What have you been doing differently to move? Dancing? Walking? Riding a bike? All these are measurable as you get stronger and can move more vigorously and for longer periods of time.
6. How are you sleeping? Using the declarations will assist in better sleep. Repeating them at bedtime, or if you wake during the night let your mind know that it is time to relax.
7. Do you feel happy for no particular

reason? Do you notice that in general you feel better? That's measurable

8. Do you notice that people are treating you differently? As you allow your light to shine you unconsciously give others permission to do the same.
9. Patience. Noticing yourself being more patient with family, co-workers, friends? As you continue practicing you will find that what used to bother you – just doesn't anymore.
10. And finally, notice how much more patient and kinder you are to yourself. As you reignite your own internal light and keep that connection with your Higher Power current, fresh and continuous you will find life much easier and joyful.

As you continue to succeed, you are building the muscle of a new lifestyle, and as we all know the more you use a muscle the stronger it gets. I know you probably are already saying to yourself "yeah but," so in the next chapter we will look at some of the many obstacles that may or may not come up for you.

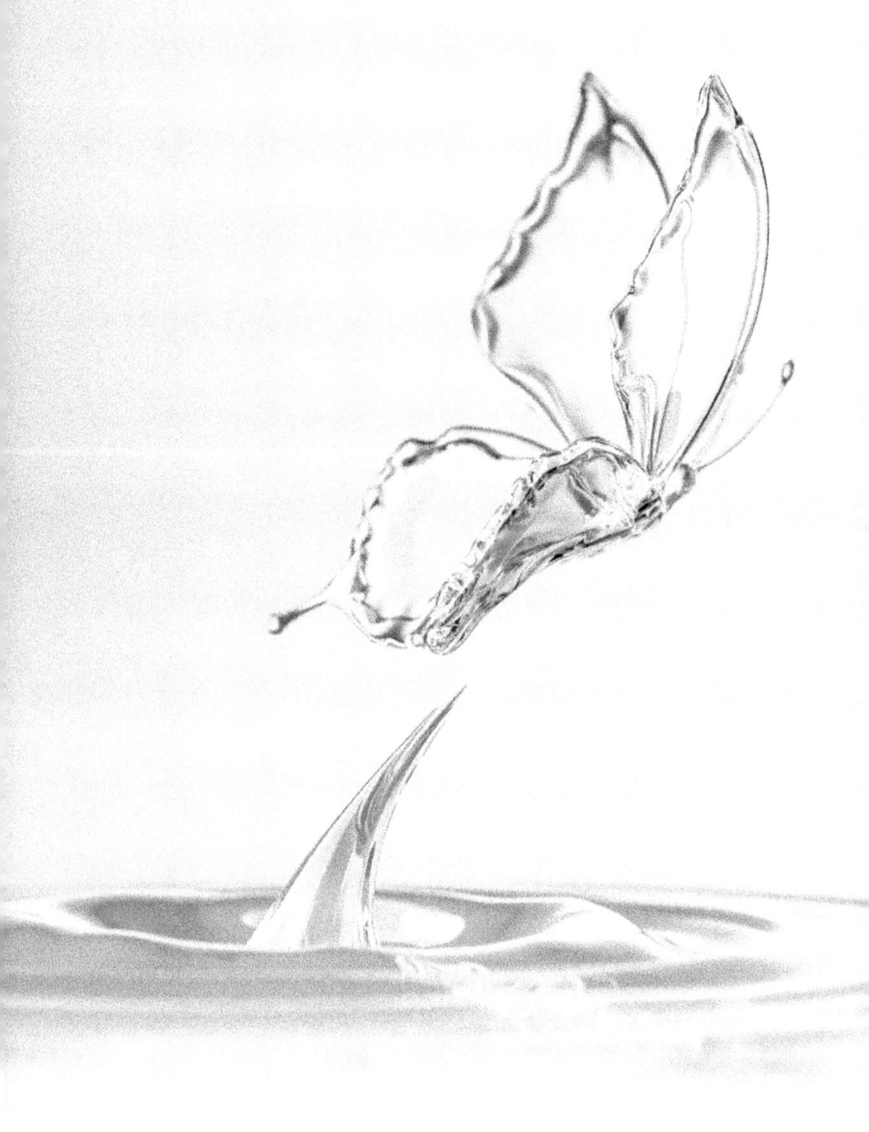

12

THAT ALL SOUNDS GREAT, BUT WHAT ABOUT...

Gina's greatest fear was that just like so many other programs this would not work long-term. She really doubted that this could be any different than what she had done before until she started working with me and her Higher Power as a partner. She had never had the knowledge she learned in this process to enable her to make the food choices with understanding and allow her Higher Power to be a partner in her process.

In the past, there had been cheat days that turned into cheat months because she was relying on her own willpower and did not understand her inner four-year-old. She learned to have compassion for her inner four-year-old, love her and walk away. Courage.

You will find there are food sabotages in your life that bring you foods "to make you feel better" that really will make you feel worse. As you practice the techniques you learn here you will find that your resistance muscle gets stronger. I can teach you a new language: how to respond to those who you think will be hurt by your refusing to eat the foods they bring. Would you give poison to your best friend? Are they really your friends if they don't respect your health and well-being? One great way to avoid those goodies that someone made "just for you" is to take one or two bites. State that you are really not hungry or so full and ask if you can take it home. Once home it goes in the waste because if it does not it goes around your waist. Where would you rather have it? In the waste or around your waist? Either way it is waste.

The smell of a doughnut literally makes my lips curl in disgust now. However, I used to eat them every Saturday morning. Your taste buds will change. Your desires will change. Pure sugar snacks or candies literally make my stomach burn now because my gut flora is healthy and does not like sugar. This can happen for you, too! Remember a craving is only a thought and now you have control of your thoughts. They pass.

There will be the treats at the office that look so delicious. The candy jar that seems to taunt your every time you walk by.

Those stressful days when you just want your "comfort foods."

Holidays will come around "with all my favorites."

Yes, there will be many things that can be obstacles. But if you continue to practice what you learned in this book you will begin to gain control of your behaviors, your habits and see results that make you shine from the inside out.

I know you are probably thinking, "How is this going to be any different than all the things I have tried before?" The real difference here is the understanding that you are not alone in this journey. When you really begin to connect with your Higher Power you are literally boosting your success. Success on steroids so to speak! Yes, this will take time and effort on your behalf just as anything worthwhile does. I hope you wear this book out by rereading the techniques, understanding the physiology of your body, remembering and using the declarations. This is a process. One that has been proven in our clinic for hundreds of clients. The ones that are the most successful are the ones that practice daily, really take seriously what they are putting in their mouth and having a support system with a family member, friend, coach, etcetera.

Your brain has the capacity to change its thoughts, habits, and behaviors. You are the manager of your brain. You can do this. And you are not alone. Be patient with yourself and trust the process. Trust your Higher Power. Trust your heart. Your inner teacher.

Visualization is a powerful tool as we have discussed earlier. Train your brain by running the success movie often. Teach it to feel the success of your progress and know that it is completely possible.

Yes, you will be tempted and may stumble. We all do. Just remember it is not the end of the world. We want to enjoy our lives and sometimes this will include an indulgence or two. Nothing wrong with that. Slow down and enjoy the indulgence as a choice you are making and get back into a healthy eating pattern right after. I love gelato and when I have it I savor each bite! You will also begin to find ways of enjoying foods differently. There are healthy options of delicious foods and treats. Google is our friend when looking for things that taste great and can be much healthier options. For instance check out AllDayIDreamAboutFood.com for amazing healthy alternatives for cakes, cookies, etcetera. Just remember that eating to try to get through something stressful or a feeling you don't necessarily like will not make it better. Find something more satisfying than putting something in your mouth to do. Call a friend, go for a walk, watch a funny TV show. Fainting goat videos are hilarious! So are kitten videos. The desire to put something in your mouth for comfort will pass! Give it five minutes and see what happens.

Okay, Let's Do This!

Whenever an obstacle comes up, revisit the techniques, practices, brain hacks, and declarations shared in this book. The chapters are not long and are there to help you assist yourself in remembering and using the techniques. I recommend you read the whole chapter as you search for the practices.

Stress reduction and elimination techniques can be found in Chapter 6. There you will find the easy and simple practices to try, memorize and carry with you.

Chapter 7 discusses HeartMath™ and Heart

Breathing™ and the coherence of brain, gut, and heart.

Refresh your knowledge of how to *Toss the Thought* is in Chapter 8. This technique is an excellent way to gain control of your negative thoughts and quickly change them to supportive positive energy by reframing and adding emotion.

Chapter 9 is where you can locate the declarations, how to begin to use them, and best practices

And the icing on the cake: your future progression visualization to really cement into your subconscious mind the delicious success of your future. Revisit Chapter 10.

My wish for you is that the information in this book will help you to understand how what you are eating, thinking, and feeling all contribute to your overall health. Through the many years I have worked with clients, I discovered it is not about the "diet" you are on but the process of really living from the inside out, living a life where joy is part of your vocabulary. As you practice the techniques here your inner light will return. It has always been there. It just has dimmed a bit and now it is time to re-ignite your life. Really find true happiness, wonder and joy that is always available to you. I'm excited for you!

There, of course, is much more. Additional declarations are available, and I do work virtually one-on-one as well. I am a public speaker and love to share this information with groups. I have a YouTube channel with additional helpful videos and my website is PamLeno.com and WeightLossHypnosisBook.com.

I would love to hear from you. You can reach me through my website and leave a comment, brag about your success, and more. I **love** you all. Cheers!

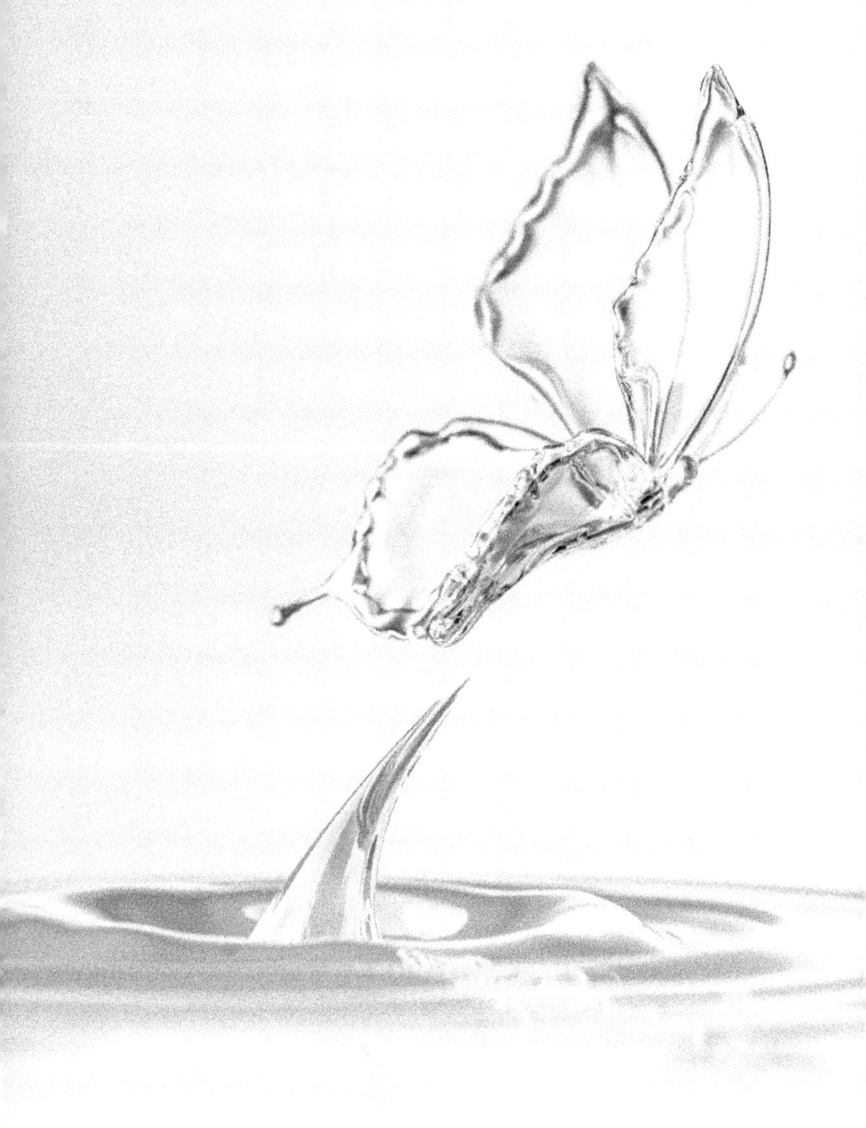

ACKNOWLEDGMENTS

This book has been a process of learning, experience, and faith. Years of working with clients, experiencing their success, and building my faith in my Divine lead to the inspiration to write this book and share it with you today.

I am deeply grateful to Angela Lauria and the staff at The Author Incubator for believing in this idea and providing me the building blocks and deadlines to keep me moving forward. You are all rock stars and are contributing to the well-being of our planet!

To my secret mentors, Marianne Williamson, Wayne Dyer, Byron Katie, Neal Donald Walsh, Elizabeth Gilbert, and Mike Dooley. Your inspiration as authors and thought leaders changed my life. I refer my clients to your work constantly and I would not be where I am today without your work in my life.

I especially want to thank Erika Flint and Calvin Banyan for being the best hypnotherapy instructors I know and for teaching me the art of self-hypnosis and the belief and strength of my Higher Power.

To my children, Chelsea Anna Marie and Sean Burns, you are my shining stars.

To my sisters, Kathy Wolf and Cindy Basso, thank you for always being by my side through thick and thin. I so appreciate your belief in me.

To my staff and clients at Ideal Wellness NW, thank you for providing much of the material in this book. Jacqui, Jody, Valerie, and Ashley, I couldn't have done this without your help in the office. You all have taught me more over the last many years than I have ever taught you. You continue to inspire me.

And to my love, Bob, my rib. Thank you for being my best friend and companion. I am so grateful for you. You have always believed in me and supported me. There are no words.

And finally, my Divine. Through the connection I now have with You and the power You bestow in me supersedes anything I could ever have considered possible. You are the true author of this book. I, only Your scribe.

ABOUT THE AUTHOR

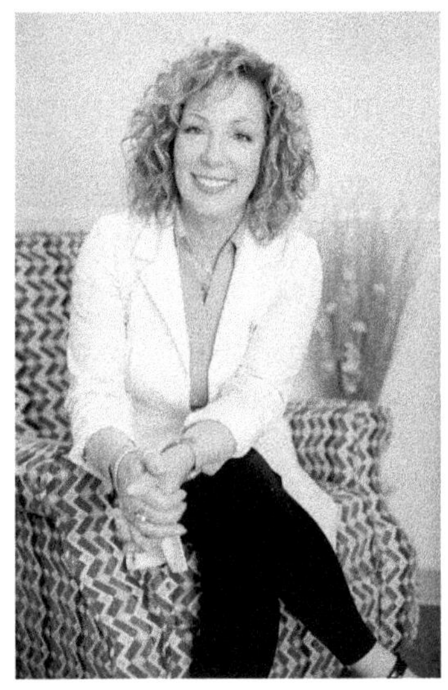

Pamela J. Leno is the owner and founder of Ideal Wellness NW in Olympia, Washington. She is a mother, author, speaker, teacher, certified master hypnotherapist, and certified life coach. In her pursuit of healthy living and helping people achieve their physical, mental, and spiritual goals, she has taken on many different roles.

After thirty years in the fitness industry, Pam realized that exercise is great for general health, wellbeing, and feeling good, but not the best option to lose weight. In 2011, she joined forces with Dr. Robert Nooney to investigate how the foods we eat actually affect not only weight but mental, physical, and hormonal balance.

Pam learned more about nutrition and hormonal imbalance during this time than she had ever learned in her years as a fitness coach.

She began to understand that there were underlying thoughts, feelings, beliefs, experiences that her clients just could not get beyond. She obtained her QSCA Coaching Certificate in 2015 and then studied under Brendon Burchard for HPC. Next was the QEHI Hypnotherapy Mastery Certification and her favorite 5-PATH and 7th Path Master Hypnotherapist Certification and Self Hypnosis Certification. She is a member of the National Guild of Hypnotherapists.

She has devoted the last ten years to learning not just the physical outcomes of poor eating habits but the emotional and spiritual outcomes of unhealthy eating habits, personal neglect, and lack of spiritual connection.

Pam loves nature. That is her church. She lives in Olympia, Washington, on Summit Lake. Nature and water rejuvenate her. She is grateful for life, health, and vitality, and wishes the same to all.

ABOUT DIFFERENCE PRESS

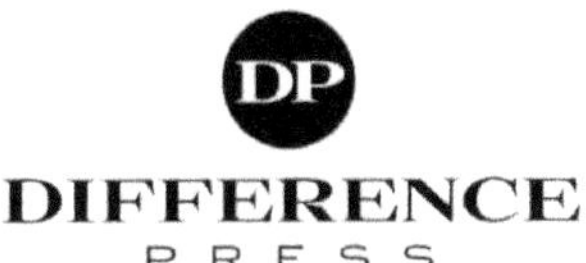

Difference Press is the exclusive publishing arm of The Author Incubator, an educational company for entrepreneurs – including life coaches, healers, consultants, and community leaders – looking for a comprehensive solution to get their books written, published, and promoted. Its founder, Dr. Angela Lauria, has been bringing to life the literary ventures of hundreds of authors-in-transformation since 1994.

A boutique-style self-publishing service for clients of The Author Incubator, Difference Press boasts a fair and easy-to-understand profit structure, low-priced author copies, and author-friendly contract terms. Most importantly, all of our #incubatedauthors maintain ownership of their copyright at all times.

LET'S START A MOVEMENT WITH YOUR MESSAGE

In a market where hundreds of thousands of books are published every year and are never heard from again, The Author Incubator is different. Not only do all Difference Press books reach Amazon bestseller status, but all of our authors are actively changing lives and making a difference.

Since launching in 2013, we've served over 500 authors who came to us with an idea for a book and were able to write it and get it self-published in less than 6 months. In addition, more than 100 of those books were picked up by traditional publishers and are now available in bookstores. We do this by selecting the highest quality and highest potential applicants for our future programs.

Our program doesn't only teach you how to write a book – our team of coaches, developmental editors, copy editors, art directors, and marketing experts incubate you from having a book idea to being a published, bestselling author, ensuring that the book you create can actually make a difference in the world. Then we give you the training you need to use your book to make the difference in the world, or to create a business out of serving your readers.

ARE YOU READY TO MAKE A DIFFERENCE?

You've seen other people make a difference with a book. Now it's your turn. If you are ready to stop watching and start taking massive action, go to http://theauthorincubator.com/apply/.

"Yes, I'm ready!"

OTHER BOOKS BY DIFFERENCE PRESS

Break the Cycle with Your Mother: Best Practices When Your Past Stands in the Way of Your Success by Christine Crise

Improve Your Health with Foundational Medicine: Avoid Drugs by Only Using Herbs and Treatments to Strengthen the Body by Terry D. Hug

Live Life Beautifully (With a Little Help): Skin Secrets for Healthy Aging to Look and Feel Your Best at Any Age by Kristen M. Jacobs, M.D.

Suicidal Thoughts and You: Escaping the Mental Loop of Wanting to End it All by Ashley McKenna, LPCC

The Dad Dilemma: How to Heal the Relationship with Your Father and Stop Recreating this Dynamic in Other Relationships by Maria Moellenberg, MA, LMFT

The Confident Grief Coach: A Guide for Helping Clients Process Loss by Patricia Sheveland

THANK YOU

Thank you for reading this book. I am beyond grateful for the trust you bestowed upon me in guiding you on this journey toward your healthier, slimmer, joyful self.

I hope you found the answers you were looking for. For those of you who'd like to learn more and continue this conversation with me, please go to PamLeno.com. Let me know how you are doing. For audio recordings to support of this book and stress relief, better sleep, and your future progression visualization practice go to WeightLossHypnosis-Book.com.

With love,
Pamela Leno

www.ingramcontent.com/pod-product-compliance
Ingram Content Group UK Ltd.
Pitfield, Milton Keynes, MK11 3LW, UK
UKHW021936190726
13853UKWH00004B/1475

9 798495 529885